"A groundbreaking integration of positive psy[chology] Erica's book provides just the right mix of p[ractical] heart-opening compassion. You will find the \ telling is both provoking and healing. I recommend this book for everyone looking to truly love their bodies."

—**Kino MacGregor**, author, yoga teacher, speaker,
and founder of Omstars

"I'm proud of Erica Mather's contribution to humanity as a Forrest Yoga Guardian, and now as an author. Erica's book, *Your Body, Your Best Friend*, holds the keys to freedom from your mental imprisonment. Erica's deeply intelligent investigation into the nature of entrapment is fascinating. Breathe deeply as you read. Seek out these keys and take action. Good hunting!"

—**Ana Tiger Forrest**, creatrix of Forrest Yoga,
and author of *Fierce Medicine*

"Erica is a true 'body whisperer,' helping women to create a truly healthy relationship with their bodies. Erica is one of my favorite yoga teachers, and I've always found her compassion and genuine love of humans allows me to return to center, and integrate body and heart. May this book touch many women with its vulnerable wisdom and powerful truths."

—**HeatherAsh Amara**, author of *Warrior Goddess Training*
and *The Warrior Heart Practice*

"Informative, honest, and free of judgment, Erica Mather's book can help even the most self-critical of us to view our bodies in an uplifting light. *Your Body, Your Best Friend* is exactly what our society needs more of: a break-down of where we've gone wrong in how we relate to our bodies, and the guidance to get it right."

—**Ariane Resnick, CNC**, chef, author, and wellness expert

"Grounded yet mystical, Erica Mather brings both practical advice and nourishing wisdom to help you create a healthy, heartfelt relationship to your body. Trading comparisons for compassion and perfectionism for potential, in these pages you'll learn to tend to your body with more creativity and lasting kindness."

—**Elena Brower**, author of *Practice You*

"Erica Mather has written a masterpiece! Even if you've digested a library full of diet, exercise, spirituality, and self-help books, you've never heard (or even thought) of the life-changing concepts in this book. This wise and inspiring manual for making your body your best friend comes from a woman you will want as your other best friend. She's *that* special."

—**Linda Sivertsen**, author, and host of the *Beautiful Writers Podcast*

"This book is everything! For a start, Erica reminds us that we are not alone in our body confusion. She teaches us why this has happened with smarts and clarity that allow us to feel smart, too. Then she empowers us through meditations, journaling, and sensory awakenings that help us find our way home again—home to our own, good bodies that are just the right size to hold all the love and pain and beauty of a real life. I'm giving this book to all my women friends."

—**Cyndi Lee**, founder of, OM Yoga, and author of *Yoga Body, Buddha Mind* and *May I Be Happy*

"With *Your Body, Your Best Friend*, Erica Mather has created a road map on how to interrupt conversations that make us feel unworthy. It's mystical, spiritual, practical, but mostly: truthful. This is a book I'll be buying for all the women in my life."

—**Jennifer Pastiloff**, author of *On Being Human*

"*Your Body, Your Best Friend* is the ultimate guide for how to feel amazing in your own skin. Erica skillfully inspires and prompts you to shed the habitual behaviors, obsessive thoughts, and negative self-talk that can get in the way of compassion, love, and joy. She makes radical acceptance accessible."

—**Tasha Eichenseher**, former brand director at *Yoga Journal*, and yoga teacher

"Erica Mather is living evidence that your body can be your best friend. She has tirelessly done the work, and is the perfect leader for anyone who is willing to change and heal the way they connect with themselves. This potentially life-changing read will guide you to see and experience yourself in a new and exciting way. These pages contain medicine that reaches deep into the body, mind, and soul."

—**Kyle Gray**, author of *Raise Your Vibration* and *Angel Numbers*

YOUR BODY, YOUR BEST FRIEND

End *the* **Confidence-Crushing Pursuit** *of* **Unrealistic Beauty Standards** **& Embrace Your True Power**

ERICA MATHER

REVEAL PRESS

AN IMPRINT OF NEW HARBINGER PUBLICATIONS

Publisher's Note

This publication is designed to provide accurate and authoritative information in regard to the subject matter covered. It is sold with the understanding that the publisher is not engaged in rendering psychological, financial, legal, or other professional services. If expert assistance or counseling is needed, the services of a competent professional should be sought.

In consideration of evolving American English usage standards, and reflecting a commitment to equity for all genders, "they/them" may be used in this book to denote singular persons.

Distributed in Canada by Raincoast Books

Copyright © 2020 by Erica Mather
New Harbinger Publications, Inc.
5674 Shattuck Avenue
Oakland, CA 94609
www.newharbinger.com

Cover design by Amy Daniel; Acquired by Ryan Buresh;
Edited by Kristi Hein

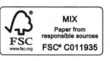

MIX
Paper from
responsible sources
FSC® C011935

Library of Congress Cataloging-in-Publication Data

Names: Mather, Erica, author.
Title: Your body, your best friend / Erica Mather.
Description: Oakland, CA : New Harbinger Publications, [2020] | Includes bibliographical references.
Identifiers: LCCN 2019054110 (print) | LCCN 2019054111 (ebook) | ISBN 9781684033430 (paperback) | ISBN 9781684033447 (pdf) | ISBN 9781684033454 (epub)
Subjects: LCSH: Body image. | Body image in women. | Self-acceptance.
Classification: LCC BF697.5.B63 M385 2020 (print) | LCC BF697.5.B63 (ebook) | DDC 306.4/613--dc23
LC record available at https://lccn.loc.gov/2019054110
LC ebook record available at https://lccn.loc.gov/2019054111

Printed in the United States of America

22   21   20

10   9   8   7   6   5   4   3   2   1   First Printing

To all the women of the past, present, and future who dare turn their suffering into great wisdom and beauty.

The body is the shore on the ocean of being.

—Sufi (anonymous)

Contents

Introduction

Hello, dear reader! Congratulations! I hope that this will be the most important book you ever read. Yes! That is my wish for you.

Why? Because I have a deeply held belief that our relationship with our bodies is the most crucial relationship of our lives. You might scoff, but consider this—it is your *primary* relationship, the one that will be with you until you die. Relating with the body is the training ground for learning the most noble of human qualities: understanding, patience, compassion, generosity, acceptance, and appreciation, to name a few. In essence, many of the energies that make up what we call "love."

Beyond this, I also believe that we humans (women, in particular, but also men) spend entirely too much time doing battle with our bodies, hating our bodies, and trying to change our bodies in impossible ways. It is—mostly—time wasted. It's precious minutes, hours, *days* we could be putting to much greater use, for ourselves, the people we love, society, and the planet.

It might be selfish of me, but I want to reap the rewards of *you* spending less time worrying about a thigh gap and more time thinking about improving air quality. Or whatever is your passion. Silly, selfish me! If this book can affect the way you think about your body, it will indeed be the most revolutionary book you *ever read*. It could change your life, and mine! This is my sincerest hope.

You might wonder what authority I have to write this book. Well, first, I'm a human with a body. But beyond that, there are two main narrative strands that have led me to this concern for the time we waste hating our bodies.

First, I've struggled with body-image distortion my entire life. I've learned from my challenges with emotional overeating, restricting, and compulsive overexercising to come into a different relationship with my body and the being living within. The primary tools I've used along the way and that I will teach you about are yoga (specifically Forrest Yoga, a yoga method in which I am a "Guardian" or high-ranking senior teacher/teacher trainer) and Buddhism. Therapy has also figured hugely into my recovery, but I'm unqualified to instruct you in that area.

Second, I've been living with chronic injury and illness for nearly thirty years. Childhood athletics and professional piano playing damaged my body in ways I'll never recover from. Adult-onset migraines were what finally broke me completely, brought me to yoga, and taught me to create this new relationship with my body and the pain it feels. So much of my knowledge and wisdom has come through engaging with my own injury and illness, using the tools of yoga, and then applying them to many hundreds of yoga students in New York City.

Along the way, I've established a business called The Yoga Clinic, which focuses on the therapeutic applications of yoga for people who are challenged by injury, illness, and aging. I've also founded a coaching program, the Adore Your Body Transformational Program, which helps people overcome their challenges with body image. In addition to working on myself, I've worked with hundreds (perhaps thousands by now!) of bodies over my fifteen years of teaching yoga full time in New York City. The wisdom that I've generated for myself I've also shared with others, and I've had the honor and privilege to witness its effects.

Long ago I learned from my teacher Ana Forrest that as yoga teachers part of our sacred task is to transform the difficulties of our own lives into wisdom for our students, to help get them out of suffering. My body-image challenges and chronic illness are the mud from which have sprung the lotus flowers of my healing work and helpful offering. *No mud; no lotus.*

I believe myself to be a success story of sorts. My students tend to agree. The transformation of my own suffering into wisdom for others has been impactful for them.

Along the way, as I deliberately engaged the issue of body image, I swiftly realized it's an intersectional issue. It stands at the crossroads of so many "isms": ageism, ableism, sizeism, racism, sexism and heterosexism. And, of course, fatphobia. As a white, middleclass, cisgendered, curvy, attractive, and straight woman, I cannot speak for any marginalized group. Mine is decidedly a voice from a place of privilege. Still, I hope that as an allied force, I am able to move the needle on the conversation.

There's never been a better time to learn to love the bodies we're in. Writers and artists, healers and activists—many of them women, many of them people of color—are rejecting body shame and embracing body positivity. When myths and cultural ideas hurt us and make us feel bad about our bodies, we're insisting on the real truth: that every body is sacred and amazing, and that real beauty follows no rules. My life's work, including this book, is my contribution to this conversation, and I hope you'll find inspiration here. Some of my favorite voices in the body-love choir are listed in the back of this book. If you leave this book ready to find more ways to own your beauty and adore your body, check them out.

I'm interested in the life of the mind and how it interacts with our bodies, and vice versa, contributing to (or detracting from) our health. As such, this book is primarily spiritual and philosophical, intended to inform the reader about the foibles intrinsic to the human species, the invisible forces and expectations humans have created for them¬selves through a collective effort called "society," and to suggest how we can resist those forces and reshape them. My mission is to help people feel better in and about their bodies, whether through group or private yoga practice, or through changing your mind, which is what I hope this book will accomplish for you.

Because I am writing as an American, the vantage point of this book is also decidedly American, with all the complexity therein. Our body-image challenges are tempered by our cultural norms, as well as the body into which we've been born. For example, at a housewarming party in Brooklyn while I was telling a fellow reveler about this book she swiftly chastened me: "I'm Latina, and we don't have the kind of body-image problems white people do! We *celebrate* our bodies!" How appearances can be deceiving! I myself am an example of this phenomenon. Though I present and identify as White, I had an abuela, my father was a first-generation bilingual immigrant, and I have a sprawling Puerto Rican family (It's best not to judge a book by its cover!). But Latina heritage didn't shield me from American beauty standards. Moreover, many of my Latinx friends in New York and beyond report that their culture is even *more* vicious about beauty standards than "normalized" American ideals. There are many cultural variances within this vast nation, and this book specifically addresses the unrealistic beauty standards to which many American women are held. However, American beauty standards have been exported around the world and impact many outside of the US. It is my hope that everyone can find some useful skill, tool, or insight within this book.

We reside within the context of our culture as both the object and the subject of our experiences. When I told a guy friend about this book, he exclaimed, "*You*?! Body-image challenges? But you're *gorgeous.*" He found it impossible to comprehend that people *he finds attractive* may not find themselves attractive. My research has shown me that the exterior of a person may or may not relate congruently to their real lived experience, their impressions of themselves, how others see them, and how they present themselves to the world. "Beautiful" people may believe themselves to be ugly. A "less socially acceptable looking" person may radiate confidence and therefore exude beauty. The axiom is true: *you cannot judge a book by its cover.* The inner workings of a person's mind may or may not match their exterior. This book will also look at how humans work, as individuals, and help you, the reader, handle your human nature to your advantage.

To accomplish these goals, in each chapter, I will identify a harmful mind-set humans are prone to perpetuating, show how that is enforced through historical precedent and modern social forces, how you as an individual cooperate with realities that harm you, and ultimately offer solutions for how to change it. Embedded within each chapter you will also find tips, practices, and exercises to help support the overarching project. You'll probably want to have a notebook or a journal by your side as you read, so you can be prepared to engage with the exercises as they appear. Or, if you prefer, you can download all of the journal prompts (and other resources) at http://www .newharbinger.com/43430.

Finally, at the end of each chapter you will find a main core practice that I've recognized as concrete enough, and important enough, that I think it's a crucial building block for creating a better relationship with your body and therefore a more satisfying life. Every chapter introduces you to what one of my clients recognized as a "replacement mind-set." We're going to "uninstall" the habitual mind-sets that harm you and replace them with new ways of thinking designed to help you.

Does that sound intriguing to you? I hope so! The promise of this book is that you will emancipate your mind so that your body also is free—and becomes the main instrument and ally through which you discover and activate your own highest good. Let's get started!

Disarm the Happiness Trap

Long before the modern pressures we now experience via social media, I grew up in the 1980s examining *Victoria's Secret* underwear catalogs for signs of how I "ought to be." I recall experiencing a complex mixture of self-loathing for my failures, envy for the beauty the magazine models possessed, and a bright ember of enthusiasm for all the ways that I was going to become slim and sexy. As a tall, busty brunette growing up in the Midwest, those aspirations seemed both surprisingly attainable (maybe if I lost 10 pounds) and hopelessly far-fetched (oh, but there is no way to alter the bone structure of my hips!).

My body-image distortion had begun years in advance of that glossy catalog and its pretty teenage models catching my eye, yet so many of my thoughts and emotions crystallized around its pages.

I thought (in no particular order):

- My life will be better when I'm thin.

- No wonder the boys don't like me—I'm not sexy enough!

- Those women are so beautiful—I know that their lives must be amazing. They must be so happy. They must be loved.

- They must have amazing sex.

- I wonder if I'll ever be desirable enough to have sex.

I'd check the mirror to see if anything had improved.

Nope. Not yet. Keep working out, eating less, dreaming, hoping; one day you'll be worthy of a good life, worthy of experiencing love…

The Buddhist Vietnamese writer and teacher Thích Nhất Hạnh says, when the present moment is simply too difficult to bear, hope is a strategy for people to differ their lives into a future, better time.[1] Young Erica became an expert at differing.

My youthful inner ecology was painful and confusing. It's difficult being a teenager! We'd rather live outside ourselves and project externally rather than go within and feel. Looking at the catalogs kept me outside of myself and helped me envision a course of action I could anticipate with excitement: the future me would be slim, sexy, happy, loved, and successful. The present moment felt too difficult to bear, so I clung to hope.

I went to the gym and worked on this self-improvement project. I ate in ways that I *thought* would support the better future me, by dieting. Ten years later, my friend Ann wailed "You're toooooooo thin!" Well...what a surprise! It simply never occurred to me that being *too thin* was even *possible* for someone like me; I thought I was doomed to be eternally tall and fat. I'd overshot the mark!? But I respected Ann's opinion, so I took it to heart and took stock. What had I actually achieved by becoming thin? Had I met my life goals? The answer was mostly *no*. Though I felt accomplished being thin, the happiness, success, and love that I expected to experience once skinny eluded me still.

Nevertheless, I thought the burden of fault was entirely mine. Clearly, if I wasn't happy even as a thin person, I was doing it wrong. Of one thing I was absolutely sure: there must exist some magic, secret mystery that everyone else knew about and allowed them to "get it right." Once I discovered it, I too would finally be cleansed of the stain of unworthiness, welcomed into the happiness club, and elevated in life. Happy at last! Happy at last! Happy at last!

I persisted with seeking happiness outside, instead of within.

Can you relate? Have you fallen into this trap? It's tragic how our culture compels us to look in all the wrong places for all the wrong things. Surrounded by its messages dictating what happiness is and isn't (and how to get it), we've become so desperately estranged from ourselves that we've impaired our ability to recognize what yields real happiness. We're consuming empty calories and expecting to feel nourished. No wonder we're so starved for true happiness.

A NATIONAL OBSESSION THAT'S MAKING US MISERABLE

Our ideals about happiness are culturally loaded. We live in a society positively obsessed with the idea that certain things will make you happy. The right job, the right clothes, a great body, a beautiful face, a pleasing partner, an amazing love life—*these* are essential ingredients for a happy life, or so we're repeatedly told.

Happiness is such an important part of American national identity that it's written into the Declaration of Independence: "We hold these truths to be self-evident, that all men are created equal, that they are endowed by their Creator with certain unalienable Rights, that among these are Life, Liberty and the pursuit of Happiness."

Our right to happiness is baked into the DNA of the United States, our collective consciousness, and therefore the collective awareness of all the countries that America affects. As we are the primary exporter of culture around the world, these concepts impact practically the entire planet.

"Happiness" is a curious principle to emphasize, since it's never been the pressing concern of any major religion or philosophical study, and our country was founded essentially on the beliefs of men who self-identified as Christians. What did they mean?

It was Thomas Jefferson who declared that the pursuit of happiness was an inalienable right, along with life and liberty. "The story goes that Jefferson, on the advice of Benjamin Franklin, substituted the phrase "'pursuit of happiness'" for the word "'property,'" which was favored by George Mason. Franklin thought that "'property'" was too narrow a notion."[2] Did our Founding Fathers believe that having property and happiness were synonymous? Or that possession of property *leads* to happiness? Certainly, the central tension in the United States is about whether the interests of the individual, business, and government can coincide, or if they're at odds. Free-market capitalists will state that regulation impedes the liberty of business, which is, at its core, a collective of people. More socially liberal people will point out that our collective caring for people is part of what makes us happy. Either way it's all lofty thinking, because happiness isn't an ideological construct: it's a feeling experienced in the body. When we ignore, deny, or abuse the body, we're not setting the stage for happiness to occur.

Work creates capital (money), which allows for the possession of property. Work is, mostly, completed by people, and people have bodies. Does it matter if people have possessions if their daily experience of work is oppressive to their bodies, minds, and spirits? It does. When individuals are unhappy, they create unhappy businesses, governments, and societies. Society isn't an abstraction: it's created by the thoughts, speech, and actions of individuals and groups of people.

You are society.

For most of us, work, accomplished with our bodies—even if it's just sitting in a chair and tapping our fingers on electronic devices—comprises the majority of how we spend our time. How many hours a day do you spend working? With so much of our lives devoted to work, clear understanding of the relationships among work, capital, possessions, and happiness helps us prudently decide how to spend the moments of our day and therefore get better, more satisfying results. Since the Founding Fathers were so deeply considering the relationship between owning property and happiness, it's no accident that we, hundreds of years later, are still wondering, and often confused, about the relationship between what we have, how we acquire it, and how (un)happy we are.

Society isn't an abstraction: it's created by the thoughts, speech, and actions of individuals and groups of people.

When you know who and what you are, you're more likely to contribute fully to the world though work, service, or art. This notion is grounded in another American ideal. President Kennedy believed that happiness stemmed from "the full use of one's talents along the lines of excellence."[3] It's not hard to see how we can jump from that idea to "start a business based on the full and excellent use of your talents." It falls right in line with the American vision of self-determination, enterprise, and ingenuity. Happiness and productivity aren't merely a matter of capitalist interest, but also a spiritual concern.

So many of us have gotten far away from the inner act of finding our talents, and then exploring *how* they manifest in the world and could contribute toward the good of all. Instead, we've fallen prey to simply measuring our productivity, and the outer beauty of a body, often forgetting to evaluate whether our outer self aligns with the best aspects of our inner self.

What might be some more reliable external indicators of happiness? Gallup Inc. asked around 1,000 people in each of 148 countries if they were well rested, had been treated with respect, smiled or laughed a lot, learned or did something interesting, and felt feelings of enjoyment the previous day.[4] In Panama and Paraguay, 85 percent of those polled said yes to all five, putting those countries at the top of the list. The United States ranked thirty-third in positive outlooks.

In your journal, copy down these five metrics, and rate each of these factors in your own life on a scale of 1 to 10. Title this query "Happiness Metrics."

1. Be well rested.

2. Be treated with respect.

3. Smile and laugh a lot.

4. Do something interesting.

5. Feel feelings of enjoyment.

If each one of them increased by just one numeral, what would the impact be in your life? Who would you be able to be? What would you be able to accomplish? What results could you produce?

No country has staked its identity so heavily on the externalities of happiness as the United States of America. That is, no country had until Bhutan converted their national mission to that of gross national happiness (GNH). The term "gross national happiness" was first coined by the fourth king of Bhutan, King Jigme Singye Wangchuck, in 1972 when he declared, "Gross National Happiness is more important than Gross Domestic Product." Their establishment of this mission was a direct critique of the American GDP, also known as *gross national product* (GNP), which is intended to measure national well-being—on an economic basis.

Critique of this idea of GDP came from within our own nation around the same time, when in 1968 then-presidential candidate Robert Kennedy said to the students of the University of Kansas:

> Too much and for too long, we seem to have surrendered personal excellence and community values in the mere accumulation of material things. Our gross national product, if we judge the United States of America by that, counts air pollution and cigarette advertising and ambulances to clear our highways of carnage. It counts special locks for our doors and the jails for people who break them. It counts the destruction of the redwood and the loss of our natural wonder in chaotic sprawl. It counts napalm and counts nuclear warheads and armored cars for police to fight the riots in our cities. It counts Whitman's rifle and Speck's knife and the television programs, which glorify violence in order to sell toys to our children.
>
> Yet the gross national product does not allow for the health of our children, the quality of their education, or the joy of their play. It does not include the beauty of our poetry or the strength of our marriages, the intelligence of our public debate or the integrity of our public officials. It measures neither our wit nor our courage; neither our wisdom nor our learning; neither our compassion nor our devotion to our country; it measures everything, in short, except that which makes life worthwhile. And it can tell us everything about America except why we are proud that we are Americans.[5]

Fifty years later, we're *still* missing these more meaningful measures of happiness. The trap we submit to is thinking we live in an either/or world. This is the way of the human mind. Outer *or* inner. We have a hard time holding our inner lives and outer realities together. Finding logical inconsistencies between the two, the mind reduces the world into binaries—this or that. But the human heart is capable of holding contradictions. It is able to comprehend both/and. We can have it both your way *and* mine. We can have our property *and* pursue our inner happiness as well. This notion is *spiritual capitalism*. When the people's hearts steer them correctly, they will find solutions that help others, *and* create some money along the way. Everyone wins. All boats rise.

It's not your fault that you've fallen into the "happiness trap"! You didn't invent it. It's part human nature, part social construct. The problem is, when we equate happiness with property, we begin to imagine that happiness is something material. The most material object we contact daily is our body, and as a result, we transfer notions of external happiness onto our only apparent material possession: our body.

Happiness isn't property. A fundamental error in this equation lies on both sides. We misunderstand happiness *and* we misunderstand property. *Our only true belongings are our actions.* At the end of our lives, our loved ones won't recall with admiration how thin we were. They will be talking about *who* we were, what we stood for, how we spent our lives, and how we made other people feel. *These* are the true results of our actions, our only real possessions.

Thinking about yourself, do the results and the consequences of your behavior bring you joy?

When we feel ourselves overidentifying with externalities, it can be helpful to take stock. As you gaze around your home, could you imagine your life without the objects you see? What kind of joy do they bring you? Do they please you because of their beauty, utility, or sentimental value? Is there some other reason that they inspire a feeling? What emotion is aroused, and what is its root? Would you still be happy, even if you didn't have them? Who would you be without your material possessions?

Our bodies are our primary material possession. Our health is the main pillar of our wealth. Some people lose limbs, organs, ability, or health as life progresses. Some people are born into this world without. The following exercises rely on an assumption that the body is intact, but yours might not be. If this is the case, I offer you two really juicy invitations as you do the exercise that follows:

1. Observe how your other parts have stepped up, and how they have become so smart and skilled in the absence of another. What have you gained, though absence or loss? How has your perception become heightened?

2. Find out if you can discover a deeper (perhaps even mystical!) relationship with the senses or abilities that each body part is connected to. This is the stuff of legends and superheroes. Remember the Oracle in the Matrix? Or, from more modern lore, Marvel's Daredevil? These archetypes spring from real people, and your own "superpowers" might be awaiting—should you go looking. Feel into *these* spaces, and find out where you excel and how your personal wealth has grown in unexpected ways because of your body.

To begin, shift your attention to your body. Consider your eyes and all the delight and pleasure they bring you through the gift of sight. Now, imagine for a moment your life without the ability to see. Living would be different, for sure, and also still worth it (right?), but reflect on all you see daily, or upon occasion, that brings you pleasure. Go through this exercise with all of your sensory organs.

- Eyes—What have you seen today that brings you joy?

- Ears—Imagine life without sound. Now, restore it to yourself.

- Nose—Imagine life without smell. Now, give it back.

- Tongue—Imagine life without taste! Now, restore this sense.

- Skin—Imagine life without experiencing touch. Now, return it to yourself.

I hope that you can see this exercise is meant not to depress you, but to reveal to you the happiness already available to you, courtesy of your body.

Now, let's extend this exercise to your limbs. What joy and delight do your arms and hands bring you? Think of an embrace, hanging your arm over a friend's shoulder or around their waist, helping someone with their coat, or holding a door. Our arms and hands bring us so much happiness. Consider your life without these delights. Aren't you so relieved to return to the present moment where you have them?

What pleasures do your legs and feet bring you?

I live in New York City, and breaking a foot vastly increased my appreciation for my legs and feet and the ability to go up and down stairs. This is such a basic physical ability that most of us can easily take it for granted, but what if something you wanted to do or see was at the top of a sixth-floor walkup? Being ambulatory can bring us so much pleasure, and it's so "normal" to most of us that we rarely appreciate the pleasure of walking until it is taken away. Reflect, for a moment, how your life would be different without the use (or possession!) of your legs, or feet. Now, restore this gift to yourself. *Feel how vast your appreciation is for the basic, daily, material delight of your own body.* We are already so rich, yet too often we barely perceive it.

You can continue to catalog more and more refined aspects of the body and discover what a treasure trove of joy they supply daily. Let's continue!

Title a list "Joy I Receive from My Body." Here, I'll begin:

1. *Teeth.* Allow me to chew. Radiate joy in a smile.

2. *Toe nails.* Protect the very sensitive ends of my toes, and shield the bones from being hurt. Also—they're fun to paint.

3. *Eyelashes.* Keep debris out of my eyes!

4. *Nose hairs.* Help warm the air that I breathe so it doesn't hit my lungs cold. Keep debris out of my throat and lungs. Thank you, nose hairs!

5. *You—keep going!*

6. *What else?*

7. Don't stop!

8. Three more!

9. Two more!

10. One more!

Great job. Whenever you start feeling yourself reaching outside of yourself for happiness, you can use these tools to reorient within. Remember—none of this is your fault! We've been miseducated to mess this up! These techniques are part of your new, better education.

Now let's take a deeper and a clearer look at happiness.

CORRECTING OUR MISUNDERSTANDING ABOUT HAPPINESS

Happiness is not a fixed destination where we will arrive when we *have* the things, look, experiences, or relationships we think we want. Happiness is not even a state of mind. Happiness is an emotion. Emotions occur in the body, so how we relate to our bodies affects how we experience and relate to our emotions. When we disavow our own bodies, we cut off our primary relationship in the world and the source of all our emotions, feelings, and wisdom. So sad!

It's likely that when we misunderstand the nature of *one* emotion, we also misunderstand *all* of our emotions. Not understanding our emotions—what they are, and how to respond to them—causes us tremendous suffering, and potentially even illness, which, again, affects the body.

Emotions Are Like the Weather

Sadness. Glee. Anger. Resentment. Peace. Loneliness. Contentment.

Emotions. They come, and they go. Or, they should. Sometimes, we get caught in a rut. One dreary weather pattern takes over, and all of the sudden we're experiencing internal rain showers for weeks at a time. This could just be what we call a slump, or it could turn into full-blown depression.

Buddhism understands emotions as energies of the body that proliferate through the stories the intellect perpetuates about said emotions. When we learn to work with our feelings correctly, they can be the source of our deepest wisdom.

Did you notice how the description of emotion is "energy"? A key to knowing your emotions is feeling their energies. Some modern psychologists theorize there are just six primary emotions. If you feel into your body, you'll probably easily be able to identify what each of the big six feels like through its distinctive energetic footprint.

Do this now. Shift your awareness inside. Recall the following emotions and the sensations they produce.

1. What does anger feel like, and where do you feel it in your body?

2. What does disgust feel like, and where do you feel it in your body?

3. What does fear feel like, and where do you feel it in your body?

4. What does happiness feel like, and where do you feel it in your body?

5. What does sadness feel like, and where do you feel it in your body?

6. What does surprise feel like, and where do you feel it in your body?

Each one has a track, like an animal leaving a footprint in the woods. Can you "see" that energetic footprint?

One of energy's attributes is that it likes to *move*. Built into the word "emotion" is exactly the description of energy's preferred behavior—it's "e," and motion. Movement is energy's preferred state! Emotions like to move too! Where? In your body! They must have some outlet for healthy expression. When you feel anger—where does it go? When you feel fear—where does it go? If it doesn't have an outlet, it will get stuck, warehoused somewhere in the body. Often, a backlog of trapped emotion will make us sick.

Emotions create energy in the body that must be brought to completion. Energy that's bound up or locked away possesses potential. It's lying around, just waiting to be used. When our energy gets turbid, it's like stuck weather. It makes trouble. That's why, when it rains for weeks on the East Coast, people start to react, getting cranky. Or in the Midwest, when it's over 90 degrees Fahrenheit for three weeks, people start to get irritable and angry. Of course, there are places on the planet where one weather pattern prevails, like Seattle, with its rainy fall-winter-spring, but have you noticed how when the clouds part the people who live there light up and flock to the parks, turning like sunflowers to the sun? Like Seattle, there are also people in the world who have a regular, steady, and prevailing weather cycle, and if you know them, a deviation can seem like an aberration.

The people I know who experience depression get stuck in a rut where only one kind of weather prevails. Because of this, they often imagine happiness as the exact *opposite* of their ongoing, relentless overcast skies and rainstorms—eternal sunshine. But this, too, is unnatural. The one constant of the world is change. Look around and observe nature. Change is built into everything, even something as simple as the seasons. Things that don't change are dead!

While sometimes an emotional rut is the result of a chemical imbalance, it can also be the product of our own thinking. Remember, our emotions proliferate through our thoughts. (*However:* If you suspect you have a chemical imbalance that is more deep-seated than your rainy thinking, please hear me now—*consult with your doctor.*)

Have you ever noticed how the way you think affects the way you feel?
Let's explore this now.

- Recall for a moment the worst day of your life. Just typing that instruction sent a lightning bolt through my chest! *Thoughts give your emotions prolonged life.*

- Now do this wonderful thing: spend a moment recalling the last time you really felt loved.

Just thinking about love can shift your internal chemistry and therefore the way you feel. Your thoughts are powerful instigators of your experience! If you choose your thoughts, you can affect the emotions that you experience. How cool is that?

Our thoughts and our body chemistry (which affect our emotions) are connected. Sometimes the chemistry leads to a feeling and a thought. Sometimes the thought creates the feeling and the chemistry.

And we are all individuals. Everybody has a different natural baseline internal chemistry or ecology—like a personal climate. Every body is unique. For instance, some people are born naturally cheerful. This is their first nature, their unique baseline state of being. How would you describe your own personal internal ecology? What is your relationship to that state of being?

Even people who know me are often surprised to discover that I experience, daily, massive, heartbreaking amounts of sadness. I would describe my "resting state" as sad. Part of my own personal growth path has been recognizing this as intrinsic to me and learning how to take care of my sadness in a way that is healthy and keeps my external life moving smoothly. My relationship to my sadness has matured and grown over time, to a point where I would never trade it in. It keeps me supple and open to the world.

Pause and take a moment to journal on this. Title your page "My Personal Ecology." It's really that important! How would you describe your baseline emotional ecology, and what is your relationship to it? Do you enjoy it? Do you have negative feelings about it? How does it affect your thoughts, your speech, and your behavior? Do you try to escape it? How?

Sometimes our reactions to our intrinsic nature impede our growth. For instance, I used to be ashamed of my sadness, but simultaneously I also brandished it in my art. I figured it was a great burden to the people around me, so I gave it life only within my music. While my sadness did have somewhere to live and find expression, it didn't actually *satisfy* the emotion's request. My art mostly further entrenched it. When we think that our emotions are frivolous, selfish, or burdensome, we deny ourselves the basic needs they are speaking to, and it stunts our growth and personal evolution and often makes us behave unconsciously. Look for this within yourself, and study it!

Regardless of a person's individual and basic disposition, everyone should experience gently varied emotional weather that comes and goes. When a storm or sun sticks around for too long, it spells trouble.

Our happiness is like this. It's just as unnatural to be in a constant state of happiness as it is to be in a constant state of unhappiness.

Happiness likes to move. It likes to come and go.

And so, we should let it come and go in our life, without fixating on it, without trying to get it to stick around longer than it likes.

Happiness Is Like a Cat

Ever try to herd a cat? The more you try to force the cat to stay, the more it wants to get away. I'll talk to little kids about the nature of cats.

"Do you want to know how to get the cat to come to you?"

"How?" they ask, while chasing and poking the fleeing feline.

"Leave it alone!" This ultimately brings the cat into their waiting hands. Tiny human minds blown!

If you pursue happiness with too much determination, just like a cat it will surely elude you. If you try to force it to stick around, it will absolutely scratch at the door and try to get away. Reach under the bed for it, and it will retreat. How strange is happiness' true nature!

Many research psychologists have verified happiness' cat-like nature. Put in more stark terms, the *effort* to try to feel happy can actually make us miserable.

This favorite quote from Thích Nhất Hạnh illuminates the situation. I've been living with it so long, I can't even recall where I first read it—it's been so baked into my consciousness.

> Your ability to experience happiness is in direct proportion to your ability to experience uncertainty.

What's your relationship with uncertainty?

Among the most uncertain, mysterious, and magical things in the world are our bodies! We know so little about them. One of my body-image clients realized that even if she mastered controlling her weight, the inevitable uncertainty of aging lay in wait to assail her. She reasoned, why not just get comfortable with the insecurity of it all? Lifting the burden of fearing unknowable change, she felt free to make choices that connected more clearly to her daily pleasure in living.

This path to happiness asks us to embrace the very things that make us the unhappiest. Mind you, I didn't say anything here about loving them—you have permission to go on disliking your love handles, muffin top, or thin hair. But it's crucially important we're honest with ourselves about our emotions. Truth and transformation go hand in hand.

It's worth exploring fully, writing down, even stating out loud: What is your greatest fear about your future body? Do your fears serve you?

I'm describing what's referred to as a "negative path" to happiness. It calls for us to assume a radically different stance toward what most of us spend our lives trying hard to avoid. It involves learning to enjoy uncertainty, embracing insecurity, stopping our efforts to think positively, becoming familiar with mistakes and failure, even learning to respect and value injury, illness, and death.

Many psychologists agree, that in order to be truly happy, we may actually need to be willing to experience some more negative emotions—or, at the very least, to stop running quite so hard from them. This can be a bewildering thought. It calls into question not just our methods for achieving

Truth and transformation go hand in hand.

happiness, but also our assumptions about what "happiness" really means."[6]

So we've fully established that happiness is not property, nor a destination, but it *is* an emotion, and it behaves like the weather. Then how do we generate a situation for "happiness weather"?

By *practicing* happiness.

Practicing Happiness

Here is another of my very favorite Thích Nhất Hạnh sayings: "There is no way to happiness; happiness is the way." Happiness is actually a *skill*. Skills require *practice*.

If we honestly lead our lives like this, it changes our perspective immensely. *No one can stop us from pursing our happiness.* This is a radical approach to personal responsibility, and ultimately an empowering one.

Personally, this means accepting where I am with my body—even if it's something I don't like—while simultaneously holding the space for positive change. This looks like, instead of hanging on to the skinny jeans for five years and thus feeling like a failure every time they mock us from the corner of our closet, we give them away with the hope someone will find great joy from them *today*. Buy jeans that fit and look great *now*. Trust that we will always have the resources to acquire flattering clothes that fit.

Practicing happiness now *is* happiness. If we cannot be happy with the body we have now, it's unlikely we will be happy with our "perfect" body later—the one that is subject to the forces of time and change, like injury, illness, and aging.

Buddhists call this practice "watering the seeds of happiness." When we spend our time training our thoughts to cultivate respect among the people around us, smiling, laughing, learning something new, we are watering the seeds of happiness in our minds and in our hearts.

Each and every one of us also has seeds of discontent in our minds and hearts. We water them by thinking thoughts like, *I'm so fat and disgusting! No one will ever love me.* Or *My hair is too thin. No one will ever find me attractive like this.*

There is a great saying that the yogis like to use—*what you place your attention on will grow.* Perhaps you've heard the New Age version: *what you focus on expands.* If you spend a lot of time focused on how much you hate your body, that hatred will grow. Hatred makes our bodies unhappy. For instance, if we think, *god, I'm so ugly,* our bodies hear, "I'm ugly" and therefore, we are ugly. It doesn't actually even matter whether it is true or not—we come to *believe* it. And we can choose to believe whatever we want, whether is makes sense or not.

But when we stop watering those dark, poisonous thoughts, the state of our body improves almost immediately, and we have a better chance to find relief from suffering. Water seeds of happiness in simple ways: by practicing getting enough sleep, and eating well, and spending time with people who support your highest good and who make you laugh. When our bodies are happier, our sum total is too.

Every few moments, we have a major, life-changing choice to make. Will we choose to think thoughts that water the seeds of our happiness or water our garden of dark thoughts? The choice seems so obvious, yet we go on making the wrong one repeatedly, often because we think that punishing ourselves will somehow make us better. It just doesn't work that way. No animal *really* learns anything from negative reinforcement, and the human body functions much the same. We've been trained from such a young age to treat ourselves badly—it's no wonder we are so unhappy! And when we've been invested in thinking horrible thoughts about ourselves for so long, we start to believe the lies; therefore making a different choice can feel

> *Everything is a plausible delusion.*

false. But I ask you—where has thinking our dark thoughts really gotten us? If it worked so well, wouldn't we all be much happier by now? Change is tricky, but every moment we have the biggest opportunity of a lifetime before us. Think ill of ourselves? Or think well? Which will it be? The choice is ours.

Let's make this concrete. What in your life do you have to be happy about? If a feeling of happiness is difficult to access at the moment, try this instead: What or who in your life are you grateful for? List ten things in your journal. Title your page "My Happiness List." Do this now! These are tools to help you begin to *practice happiness*.

Are Affirmations Effective?

Some people help themselves practice happiness by using affirmations, which are a category of positive thought. These might also be helpful for you. The basic notion is that positive thinking leads to more happiness; however, we also know that forced positive thinking repels happiness. With this caveat in mind, it's important how we proceed. I like to think of affirmations and all their relatives as "helpful thoughts." You can assess: *is this thought helping me or harming me?* Proceed from there.

Harmful thoughts can run the gamut from relatively benign to life-threatening. My teacher Ana Forrest calls the really bad version of self-denigrating thoughts "self-mutilation." It's the same as cutting ourselves, or beating ourselves, or otherwise harming ourselves; it just happens on the inside. But the damage is no less; in fact it might be far worse. We cut ourselves from within with our thoughts and say horrible things about our bodies. And our bodies hear us. And, since they have their own consciousness, they react.

At the other end of the spectrum from self-mutilation lies mostly a lot of insidious junk. The mind talks nonstop, and for some reason we actually pay attention to the narrative it creates. The voice in your head is rarely the best version of you. Affirmations are an effort to give yourself something useful and helpful to think when you're not really thinking about anything (junk thoughts!), or to counter a tendency toward self-mutilation. They're intended to point you, repeatedly, in the direction of your highest self.

I believe that the power of helpful thoughts is contained in three basic elements:

1. Make them yourself.

2. Ground them in truth.

3. Connect them to movement.

The uplifting thoughts that fill your head must be ones based on truth about your life, your understanding of who you are, and where you are going.

For instance, when I was recently twenty pounds heavier, I was very unhappy about it. My mind was tempted to think corrosive and abusive thoughts based on my prejudice for thinness: *You can't gain weight and teach yoga.* (*Yoga teachers are healthy people, and healthy people aren't fat! Cue all the horrible cultural health/weight biases.*) *You look so lumpy and ugly. Nothing ever goes right for you!* To indulge these notions would have meant creating a garden of dark thoughts. But to replace those thoughts with ones that were artificially positive—like "I'm becoming thinner every day!" or "I'm beautiful just the way I am!"—would have disregarded the truth of my dismay and entrenched my depression further. The soul knows when it's being duped.

Instead, I tried my best to embrace, with understanding, my disappointment, my confusion about where the weight had come from, and my disgust with the image I saw reflected in the mirror. I knew the emotions were like the weather. I understood that they would come and go. How did I know this? Because it had happened before. It's not like it was the first time I had gained weight or lost it. I had felt gross and squishy before, with my clothes not fitting right. And that time passed. And then it came back. Like the seasons, my own body fluctuates and changes. It's best to not worry about it too much and to instead focus on the important work of your life. But it's not our fault we get caught up all over again in these well-worn patterns! We've created neural pathways. They feel comfortable, like a pair of broken-in shoes. Making new pathways requires deliberate, repeated, and sustained effort.

The soul knows when it's being duped.

So what thoughts did I strive to replace the unhelpful thoughts with? Something like this: "I don't understand what is happening here, but I trust my body and it will work this out. Right now, it needs to be heavier. At other times, it will be thinner. Regardless, I will respect myself and refuse to think ill of myself and my body."

It's an affirmation I made myself based on the truth of my feelings and the situation. Here are a few other renditions of this concept, originating from different lineages.

Aspirations

For affirmations to work, they must be shot through with truth. The Buddhist nun Pema Chödrön shares some of my own critiques of them, electing a different word to describe a very specific practice in her tradition: *aspirations*. She says, "Affirmations are like telling yourself that you are compassionate and brave in order to hide the fact that secretly you feel like a loser."[7] In her tradition, the aspiration practices are linked with the Four Limitless Qualities—loving-kindness, compassion, joy, and equanimity. In her Shambhala practice it's extremely important we never try to convince ourselves that we're feeling something we're not. Instead, we must take into account the messiness of what we feel and put a beautiful spin on it, using one of these limitless qualities. You might see that the "affirmation" I just mentioned wove in compassion for my own uncomfortable predicament.

Mantra

A *mantra* is a phrase, often given to you or assigned to you by your spiritual teacher, to help you access your true nature. They're often recited in Sanskrit, a sacred language containing sounds that activate higher parts of our consciousness. Mantras aren't exactly affirmations, but they are closely related. One of my teacher friends in New York City is a very traditional yoga practitioner. He chants his mantra daily, and he told me it's become so much a part of his automatic functioning that when he's not thinking, he is thinking about his mantra. This is very useful! No more junk thoughts—only high-vibration thoughts.

Sankalpah

In yoga, we have a very specific way of crafting affirmation. We call them "intentions" or in Sanskrit, *sankalpah*.

Because yogis believe that you are everything you already need to be—there is no striving, there is nothing to fix—when we make an intention, it's always crafted in the present tense. Because it already is. We're merely uncovering the truth that lies buried. It's also stated in a positive voice, because (a little neuroscience for you here) the mind doesn't actually compute negatives. The mind works only in positive statements. For example if you say, "Don't touch the stove!" it hears "Touch the stove!" So if you are working on generating more compassion for yourself and the current weight of your body, you might say simply, "I am compassion embodied." Or if you are working on accepting the way you feel in your jeans today, "My jeans fit exactly as they should today."

As you read these examples, they are just guides for you to craft your own. You could adopt them outright, but please think first about whether you actually believe what the intention says. No point in trying to dupe yourself or try to cover up the truth about how you feel. We already know that forcing positive thinking will only take you further away from the happiness you are seeking.

Also, these examples aren't intended to encourage you to follow blindly, but for you to try on another worldview and see if it fits. This is the value of exposing yourself to other people's affirmations.

For instance, recently, I was paging through a book chock full of affirmations. Most seemed pretty silly to me, but then I came across one and had a strong, strange reaction. The affirmation was, "I get anything that I want!" The sensation that I had was of visceral recoil.

And I thought, *Well, that is a very interesting reaction. Clearly I have a charge around that one! I wonder what that is...*

That big charge got me to start workshopping *why* I had that intense, visceral response. My body told me there was something of value there to explore, and I decided to go tracking! While investigating, I generated five steps that you can use to benefit from other people's affirmations, whether you get a jolt—positive or negative!—from them or not:

1. Pull them apart to see how they work.

2. Find out what sorts of beliefs they rest on.

3. Examine those beliefs to see if they align with a vision of your best self.

4. If they contain something that you would like to build into this vision of your best self, then take the steps to do so.

5. If not, let them go or even set a boundary so this aspect can remain outside of your life.

Also, know that the thoughts we find most repellant often contain our most life-altering teachings. Stay open to everything!

Call it what you will—affirmation, mantra, sankalpah, invocation—the problem and the solution are the same: if we are left to our own devices, our minds will fill up the space inside with irrelevant, unhelpful, and perhaps even destructive thoughts. It's up to us: we can go through our lives allowing this to happen, or we can make a choice to think helpful thoughts, affirmations, aspirations, mantras, that are going to help point us in the direction of our highest good. Which will it be? The choice is yours! These helpful thoughts can be effective, and it is an interesting path to choose using them and finding out *how* they change your life.

Staying Unhappy

We've established this pretty firmly: staking our happiness on externalities such as weight or looks is almost certain to lead us *away* from the happiness we so deeply desire.

Sometimes when we start to look under the hood of our own beliefs by doing something like reading this book, and we grow, and we change, we might find out that in fact all along we were very committed to our own dead-end approach. Somehow, the way we've set things up, which we say makes us unhappy, actually serves us very well or shields us from some deeper truth or understanding that might be difficult for us to confront. You might just find that you're *committed to staying unhappy!*

Why on earth would someone want to continue to think their crappy, degrading thoughts, or believe that the only thing that makes people like them is their good looks? Here's why: the alternative is that we must take radical responsibility for our own experience, for realizing our own worth and value, for standing up for it, and making it a reality in our own lives.

That takes work.

It's far easier to feel bad about ourselves, think *why me?* and wait for other people to approve of us and our looks. I know lots of people who behave this way, and I bet you do too. One of my clients came to a sobering realization that as long as she went on believing that other people were judging her body and sizing her up as "fat," she could always ascribe every disappointment in her life to this reason. Didn't get the job? *Oh, it's because they think that I'm fat.* Didn't get the guy? *Oh, he must have thought I'm fat.* I'm not saying fat bias isn't real—it's very real indeed. But in this instance, my client came to the very brave understanding that she had been using that rationale as a shield from looking deeper into her own understanding of herself, her worth, and her belief in who and what she is and what she stands for, and from inevitably asking for more out of her life. The stakes are actually pretty high! Sometimes it's easier to stay small, play small. And that's okay, as long as you recognize what you are doing and fully accept yourself for it.

So we must always be checking in with ourselves and asking: *am I invested in staying the way I am? If so, why?* The basic reason is: on some level, it works for us. If we find out what exactly works for us, we will unearth the trap and then begin to change it. I want that freedom for you.

Ponder this for a moment: What would your life be like, and who would you be if you never again complained about your body? What if you addressed it only with expansive qualities like compassion, joy, loving-kindness, and equanimity? Sometimes when I'm asked to let go of an old, familiar habit, I can hear a tiny voice inside of me pipe up and say, *yeah, but...* Those two words *always* stall us in our forward progress. When you hear them, in your head or spoken by others, put them down. Refuse to stop at the roadblock erected by those two little words. Insist on driving off-road. Start your process of change by instead asking: *What if I could?*

When you think helpful thoughts, it positively affects your body. This is the basic, fundamental wisdom of mind-body practices.

HELPFUL THOUGHTS HAPPEN IN YOUR BODY

In the section on affirmations, I identified four basic iterations of similar ideas: affirmation, aspiration, mantra, and sankalpah. These are all what I'm calling "helpful thoughts."

There is only one place to have a thought—in your body. There is only one place to have a feeling—in your body. It's so obvious as to be ridiculous! And still we try to outmaneuver this truth at every turn.

So a skillful approach to rehabilitating our relationship with the body is to create helpful thoughts, and then to connect them to movement. When you connect your thoughts with the movement of your body, it creates a super, turbocharged kind of energy. I have an entire group of students who are engaged daily in this kind of intentional work with their yoga practices. But it doesn't have to be yoga. You could run and think your helpful thought. You could do paint or throw pots, or knit, and think your helpful thought. You could dance and think your helpful thought. The mode of movement isn't really the important part. It's the combination of movement and intentional thought that is critical.

The body's native languages are touch and movement, and when we combine them with the language of the intellect—speech—it has a potent effect on all aspects of us and deep healing potential. It's good medicine.

For this healing exercise you need two elements:

- A helpful thought

- A movement your body enjoys

This is simple and powerful, but not necessarily easy. You might need to spend some time crafting a helpful thought. If you need to, go back and review those sections for guidance.

You might need to spend even more time discovering what kind of movement your body experiences as pleasurable. Take as much time as you need! These are the crucial, foundational building blocks for the relationship of a lifetime—with your body.

SELF-DISCOVERY TAKES TIME

When my body made a last-ditch attempt to get my attention—by ruining my health with migraines—I went to see a healer. He said to me, "You are really fucked up. And if you don't start taking care of yourself, you'll be dead by the time you're forty."

Needless to say, this got my attention. I heeded his advice and started to ask, *What does it mean to take care of myself?* This question landed me in yoga class, where I found, for the very first time, movement my body actually enjoyed. I was immensely relieved, but also heartbroken, because I discovered *for the very first time* how thoroughly bereft my body had been of my time, care, and attention. No one had done this to me. I had done it to myself. Worse yet, this complete and utter self-abandonment was the result of doing what I thought was "right." Our culture teaches us to abandon ourselves, and the first, most violent act is rejecting our bodies. It's a "normal" mind-set in which many of us have become spellbound, and it's slowly killing us.

My awakening from the spell generated a lot of anger (at the world) and also regret (for how I'd harmed myself). But awakening also compelled me to keep moving forward, because moving away from a fantasy and into reality is freedom—and I *love* freedom. Not coincidentally, I think, liberty is also a founding principle of our great nation. And, dear reader, above all, I want for you your freedom. Freedom, however, is *earned.* You might recall that many wars have been fought to acquire, and defend freedom. Only when our bodies and minds are liberated are we truly free.

As of this writing, it's been eighteen years since I first took a Forrest Yoga class and began to breathe, and feel, and earn my freedom. I tell you this to put things in perspective. It all takes time. Be patient with yourself.

So far, you've already done a ton of work reframing how you think about your body and your self, and how these engage in the world. Changing your mind is the hardest thing to do, so I applaud your willingness and your efforts! Change requires not only time but also repeated effort. Sometimes students will ask me, "How long will it take to loosen my hamstrings?" or liberate some other internal barrier or painful spot they've uncovered in their body. My response generally is, "How long did it take you to make those tight hamstrings?" It's a playful question, but one designed to put into perspective our desire for a quick fix. Your body is organic. It functions on an organic schedule. Bear this in mind as you read the coming chapters. Your helpful thought and your pleasurable movement will change as you change. You'll have to pay attention, repeatedly! The entirety of what's in this book will require constant inquiry, for a lifetime. After all, you don't plant a garden once and then walk away forever. You revisit it, constantly. That said, let's continue the journey of your life.

Only when our bodies and minds are liberated are we truly free.

The Grass Is Never Greener

It's human nature to assume that others have life easier or better than us based on factors such as looks and socio-economic positioning, and often, it's true. This is the lottery of birth: we're born into bodies, families, and nations we did not choose, along with inherited advantages and disadvantages. This chapter will complicate our part in this story.

Children are especially sensitive to hierarchies of real or perceived difference and can be especially cruel to one another on this account. And, unfortunately, we often carry into adulthood wounds formed through childhood experiences.

For instance, when I returned to sixth grade from summer break, some of my "best friends" Jessie and Samantha behaved like they didn't know me. Our friendship, apparently, had come to an end.

I was heartbroken, and I didn't have the words to express it to them. Mom tried to explain away the hurt, but all my child brain really heard and remembered was, "You're different." I know that she was trying to comfort me with those words, to encourage me and help me feel better, but in my mind "different" was a horrible fate. What child longs to be different? Children want to belong and feel accepted.

But Mom said I was different, so I looked for a difference I could really see, feel, and understand. And my ten-year-old brain landed on this explanation for what had happened: *the girls who ditched me are cute, little, and blonde. I am...unusual-looking, tall, and brunette.* They sailed to popularity, while I became (in my perception) an outcast. They expelled me from their friendship circle, and the only reason I could find was the difference in our looks. My *body* was the culprit. It was to blame for my misfortune. This, I think, was the true beginning of my hatred for my body.

Certainly, it's common knowledge our culture favors those with light skin, eyes, and hair. It's entirely possible two of my elementary school friends absorbed that message and consequently felt superior to me. But honestly, I have no idea what happened to our relationship. I've never gone back to ask them, and it's doubtful I ever will have an opportunity. Anything, literally *anything* could have happened. Grown-up Erica can see that now. Jessie and Samantha did nothing to intentionally harm me.

Nonetheless, the seed was planted in my child mind. *Blonde girls don't like me, and they live charmed lives. Because they are cute, little, and blonde, people readily like accept them, and their lives are better than mine.* Do you have any ideas like this about other people?

Little Erica sought an escape from these emotional and existential traps. I figured my situation would change through association with the "right" kinds of people. Have you ever done this, or watched others do it?

I crushed on boys with radiant, societally approved looks. Their rejections devastated me—the angelic-looking yet cruel boy on swim team I had a hopeless crush on for *years*, the gang of towheaded brothers I saw only at an annual holiday party. The approval of any of them would do! I would daydream about our interactions, playing out how they would go, with me finally emerging victorious. They would see how cool I was; they'd love me, and finally I would live within the circle of their radiant blonde existence. Through the benefit of association and their approval, the charmed spell would be cast over my life as well.

This story is embarrassing to me, and I *still* feel ashamed, vulnerable, and exposed. I'd rather not admit it all; I'd really rather hide the truth, because it paints an unflattering and undignified portrait. It's a natural reaction to conceal unpleasant emotions. I'm afraid the truth might hurt people I truly care about, or perhaps even make *you*, my reader—should you fit the description of anyone in the story—anticipate judgment when we meet at a class, workshop, or retreat. I fear being misinterpreted, attacked, and misunderstood. It makes me want to press *Delete*.

This is how emotions about *difference* work. They often stay hidden, underground. They grow in strength and twist until something far, far worse emerges: hate. (Sometimes we become so blinded by our hatred we cannot recognize that the people we hate have something we desire.) All this internal and external drama develops just based on the material form of the body. It's ugly. But it's so relevant, because it reveals how something seemingly trivial, like making an assessment about your looks versus another's looks, leads to real, impactful emotional experiences that consequently affect how we behave.

The Greek philosopher Plutarch said, "Of all the disorders of the soul, envy is the one no-one confesses to."[8] Confession would admit to deeply repellent emotions. Perhaps more importantly, envy is an acknowledgment of experiencing inferiority, a self-assessment few willingly reveal. This is envy's mechanism. It stays in the shadows. Therefore it's incredibly important that we drag such unattractive emotions out and into the light, because they're at the heart of so much of what make us, and therefore, our culture, ugly.

I've told you about some of my triggers. We all have blindspots that lead us into a cascade of often erroneous assumptions about another person, who they are, and what their life is like. We've all inadvertently done this based on various biases. It's human nature. It seems like in recent years more and more people have been on the receiving end of biased treatment, too. In the moment of recognition we can make a fresh start. We can choose how we feel about ourselves and therefore relate to others, altering the kinds of experiences we have in the world and therefore the quality of life that we live. Sound like a good plan?

A CULTURE OF COMPARISON AND COMPETITION

My own envious thoughts were constructed partially from American society's preference for particular looks, and partially from my own childish invention. Children make sense of life in ways that often aren't accurate, and those inaccuracies persist into adulthood. Ana Forrest calls notions that are only sort of true—but that we take as *completely true*—"partial truths." It *is* real and true—there *are* hierarchies of power and socially conferred benefit based on what body we're born into. But our thoughts *about* that, what kind of meaning we make of it, and how we live it out in our own lives is what gives it real and true power. The whole truth is: society molds us, and we also have the power to think our own thoughts about that experience. This is the notion from which springs an adage attributed to Gandhi (and others): *Be the change you want to see in the world.*

We compare. And we make assumptions about what others think when they compare themselves to us. Concerning ourselves unnecessarily with the opinions of others, we give away our own personal power.

The general assumption goes like this: *that person's life is better than mine because (fill in the blank), and they know it, and they look down on me.*

The point of comparison is relatively arbitrary. It's the comparative assumptions that poison us. Worse yet, comparison breeds envy and resentment. Envy makes a person feel inadequate. *What I have, what I am, is not enough.* Resentment is the bitter indignation of being treated unfairly, not getting what you think you want, or being forced to do or give something against your wishes. It can come in a generality, like: *Life is not fair!!! Why was I born tall and brunette?* Or it can be aimed at a person, or group of people: *Life is not fair!! How come you are so pretty, and I am not?! I hate you!* Or *You don't look like me, so you are not as good as me.*

The logic pathway runs like this.

1. You look a certain way.

2. Therefore you have certain possessions, experiences, and relationships that result in happiness.

3. I compare myself to you.

4.   I find myself superior or inferior in different areas.

5.   I feel good where I find myself superior. Perhaps I even feel entitled to what I have. *Entitlement* is a belief that I've already earned what I have, or I don't yet have things that others are depriving me of.

6.   I feel bad about the areas where I find myself lacking.

7.   Where I feel bad, I experience envy, resentment, and perhaps greed. *Greed* means wanting what is not mine or what I have not yet earned.

8.   I want what you have. (Philosophers name "what you have" *the goods.*)

9.   I begin to behave in certain ways to prop myself up or push you down, in an effort to have what you have.

It's not pretty. This pathway gets us—individually and collectively—into a lot of trouble. And it almost *always* starts with what you look like and what kind of body you were born into.

In the end, comparative thinking is rarely helpful. *Compare and despair.* It's a mind-set we've got to dismantle!

Here's a mantra I use to handle myself: "Never begrudge others the results of their own efforts; stop comparing yourself to others, just enjoy what you have. Be your own person and appreciate what you have."[9] This is a reminder to me: I possess my own magic, and it's mostly up to me to find it, take care of it, and midwife it into the world. Getting wrapped up in envy saps our power. Wanting others' goods and not recognizing our own magic allows our magic to wither away.

Let's pause here and do a little digging into *your* life and psyche. I've shown you my ugly, ugly psyche. You don't have to show what you write down now (in your journal) to anyone except yourself, so be as candid as you possibly can. It will probably be gross, and that's okay. The transformational

Lies and transformation cannot coexist.

pathway relies on our truthfulness with ourselves, and radical acceptance of *all parts* of ourselves. Lies and transformation cannot coexist.

So be brutally honest with yourself. It's absolutely okay to feel everything that you do. The real question is, how will you respond to those feelings?

Answer these questions in your journal. Have a good cry along the way, if you need to! Get a box of tissues. Be prepared. Title your page "Envy Exposé."

1. Can you identify feelings of envy you have for other people?

2. Do you know where they came from?

3. How have they shaped your life and interactions with people?

4. In what ways have you given away your own power *to* those people?

5. Can you think of someone specific who sparks the feeling of envy within you?

6. What are some steps that you can take to make yourself feel better, in the face of that?

7. What are some steps that you can take not to harm another because you experience envy around them?

A few little questions can be so deeply upsetting!

The topic is heavy, I know. So I want to give you some tools to help lighten up, right away. Here are some tips for envy remediation.

- *When you feel envy, recognize it as a deep call from your heart.* Mama Gena of the School for the Womanly Arts advises that when you feel envy, immediately transfer it into an anticipatory excitement: recognize envy as a desire for something you do not yet have, and a sign that it is coming your way. Admire the people who possess traits and skills that you believe desirable. Seek them yourself, work for them, create the conditions for them.

- *Give yourself permission to desire.*[10] It's okay to have longings! Our transformation hinges on our honest work with the truth of our emotions.

- *Wish the best for those of whom you feel envious.*[11] It's a spiritual law: you cannot simultaneously want what someone has and resent them for having it. Resentment is repellent. You must create an inviting emotional environment. Someone's got what you want? Hot damn! Send them a prayer, and a high-five, and a "you are badass!" and praise them for all the invisible *work* that went into getting what they got. Experience what the Buddhists call "sympathetic joy." Honestly be happy for people who have what you want. Joy is attractive. Literally!

- *Assess whether you are really willing to do what it takes to have what (you think) you want.* For example, sometimes I feel envious of people who have beautiful, freestanding handstands (dorky yoga stuff, I know!). But I also am clear that I'm not willing to focus the amount of time and energy required in order to learn how to handstand sooner rather than later, if ever at all. Get clear about the costs involved in getting what you want. And, if you decide it's worth it—then get to work! Invest the time, money, and energy in acquisition of the goods.

Finally, author Robert Greene says to "accept the fact that there will be people who will surpass you in some way, and also the fact that you may envy them…let envy turn inward and it poisons the soul; expel it outward and it can move you to greater heights."[12] There is always, *always* going to be someone faster, stronger, smarter, prettier, and so on. Accepting this truth helps us move forward.

Coming to terms with ourselves and what we are in this world is the greatest work of our lives. Accepting the body is the path to the most profound self-acceptance we

Accepting the body is the path to the most profound self-acceptance we can attain in our lives.

can attain in our lives. But sometimes acceptance swings—*hard*—in the other direction.

Pathological Comparison

This obsession with comparison and competition is a problematic national pastime, *and* it's also a pretty natural human habit. Until we learn how to identify it and channel it in constructive ways, comparison simply won't bring out the best in us.

Human tendencies exist along their own spectrum. A little anxiety: normal. A lot? Trouble. A little comparison is normal. We learn to handle ourselves. If our tendency for physical comparison gains its own life, ruling us from the moment we wake up to the moment we go to sleep, it's serious. When we've crossed this line from "comparison leads to my unhappiness" to "comparison keeps me from leaving my house" (isolating), this spells trouble.

If comparison is crippling, you might suffer from a clinical disorder, called Body Dysmorphic Disorder (BDD). BDD is severely underdiagnosed, in part because clinicians are not aware of it as a diagnosis. BDD is also frequently overlooked because very often the individual feels shame—as I did—and consequently hides the actual source of concern, leading BDD to be misdiagnosed as major depressive disorder or social phobia. Here are some signs that body-image dissatisfaction deserves a deeper look and consultation with a professional.

- Belief that others take note of your appearance in a negative way.

- Avoiding social situations.

- The need to seek reassurance from others about your appearance.

  - The strong belief that you have an abnormality or defect in your appearance that makes you ugly.

  - Preoccupation with your physical appearance, with extreme self-consciousness.

- Comparison of your appearance with that of others.

  - People with BDD may examine themselves excessively or avoid mirrors altogether.

  - They may be reluctant to appear in pictures.

- The need to grow a beard or wear excessive makeup or clothing to camouflage perceived flaws.

- Excessive grooming, such as hair plucking or skin picking, or excessive exercise in an unsuccessful effort to improve the flaw.

When suffering from BDD, a person becomes so convinced the imagined flaw is real—even when it's not—that it may hinder their ability to attend school or engage in social situations. It can occupy *hours* daily, impairing the quality of life, and causing more stress than depression itself. BDD can potentially lead to heightened or more frequent thoughts of suicide.

As with most mental disorders, BDD can flare up and then go away, only to return again later. As a sufferer, I've experienced prolonged periods of calm, only to be besieged again. When I start to investigate *why now?* I'll find some other disturbance running beneath the surface. A deeper issue is bugging me, and BDD is a manifestation of a psychic irritation I'd rather not confront. Knowing this, I'm empowered to disregard the distortions I see in the mirror as mirages and illusions, and to search for what's *really* bothering me.

The tools of yoga and Buddhism have helped me, but not all people suffering from BDD may find these solutions effective. One way or another, the professionals agree that BDD does not get better over time and will not go away if you ignore it. It's best to tackle it *now*. Doctors sometimes use medications to help, and some consider cognitive behavioral therapy (CBT) effective as well. My hope is that, in addition to professional help, the tools and resources in this book will provide ongoing, daily assistance.

Mirrors, Scales, and Sizes

We do ourselves harm when we turn the destructive energies of comparison and judgment against ourselves. We stand on the scale—is the number more or less than yesterday? That little question may have inordinate power to make our day great or ruin it. A number becomes a feeling, affecting how we present ourselves, interact with others, how our day goes, and what kinds of outcomes we experience. All this from a number, how it compared to yesterday's number, and the resulting judgment brought to bear against ourselves. What a waste!

We try on a pair of pants in a store. They're not the size we'd like them to be. The mirrors are unflattering. It's a sure-fire recipe for a bad day. Worse yet—we put on a pair of pants that *used* to fit well and now they are tight, tight, tight. If you've been there, you know well how it can trigger a cascade of self-mutilating thoughts and a desperate review of the recent past for *when did I get so fat?*! Now we're comparing our present self to our past self.

We look in the mirror and see a version of ourselves. Is it different from what it was yesterday? Of course it is. Is today's version better or worse? Does it really matter? You're not the same person you were yesterday. There is no going back. And yet we expect the image we see there to be fixed. One thing we share in common for sure—we all are getting older, together. No one escapes this fact.

Reduced to a number, we transform ourselves into an object. Objectification robs us of our complexity and humanity. It's an act of violence against the self. When we do it to others, it's an act of violence against them.

We all are getting older, together.

I recall my own mother's anguish and sorrow over what she saw in the mirror. In her mind she was still twenty-six, young, thin, and beautiful. In the mirror she saw constant disappointment. It broke my heart for her that this was such an unrelenting source of suffering and unhappiness. I longed for her to have a different experience of herself, her life, her aging process. I wish she had the tools that I had found.

We use the mirror, scale, and sizes incorrectly, as a referendum of sorts. As if they can actually measure all of what we are. They can't.

The mirror plays funny tricks on us. Or do *we* play funny tricks on ourselves? Often we see things that no one else can or does see. I see aging. Others see no difference from ten years ago. I think of my mother, and I choose to relate to my aging process differently.

The mirror is the ultimate instrument of self-perception. You will usually see within it whatever is the state of your mind. Hate yourself? You'll hate what you see. Love yourself? You'll love what you see. It's a metaphor for truth.

To see, in the Buddhist sense, means to look deeply and to therefore understand. To understand means that you comprehend the ways people suffer. When you understand this, you have part of the key to relieving their suffering. This is a key element to the Buddhist practice of love, called *maitri,* and translated as "loving-kindness." When we look in the mirror, we have an opportunity to look deeply at ourselves, to understand the ways that we suffer, and to do the work for ourselves, on our own behalf, of relieving our own suffering. We can choose our thoughts about what we see.

You might have heard of Bikram yoga and some of its core elements: *heat* (107 degrees Fahrenheit!), *mirrors,* and twenty-six prescripted poses. When I tried Bikram, the presence of mirrors was intolerable. The thought of having to look at my body doing yoga for ninety minutes was more than I could endure. I asked a friend who practiced Bikram about this. She responded that it didn't bother her that much because she was instructed to look into her own eyes while she practiced, and through this she learned to see past the body and to connect with her own soul.

This is deep.

Here's a transformational exercise. Sit in front of a mirror. Set a timer for three minutes. Look yourself in the eye for those three minutes. Don't look away! Continue to gaze and find out what you see. Try looking in the left eye. Try looking in the right eye. Do this every day for thirty days! Document what you experience.

We've been trained to look in the mirror and readily accept what we think we see there as the result of all we are. Question the mirror. Dispute the assumptions you've made about what you see. If you are prone to Body Dysmorphia Disorder, *challenge* what you see. Refuse to allow it to be so simple and reductionist as to think that all you are seeing is imperfections. *Contest* the idea that all you are seeing when you look is the here and now. Can you see your past? Can you see how it is showing up in the now? Can you reach for a future version of yourself that you feel proud of?

Life is not all so material, so concrete. Reject self-objectification. Refuse to reduce yourself to something so shallow as a number or a snapshot in time. Resist allowing a weight, or a selfie, or a clothing size to be a referendum on your being. Instead, answer the call of your spirit to see the truth that everything—the past, the present, the future—is here and now and that you are infinite and eternal.

Nothing can measure the vastness of your being.

As for your scale—I think that a solid recommendation is to get rid of it. Evaluate your body based on what it feels like and what it can do. I did this for about fifteen years. Then I bought a scale. Why? Because I was curious about how the body works, and that number no longer had any power over me. A number is just a number—it has no meaning until we give it one. Take back your power from your mirror, scale, and clothing sizes.

What's Diet Culture?

We live in a diet culture. This means that our society generally accepts the idea that dieting and the desire to lose weight are virtuous and compulsory. The premise of modern day dieting is that if you work hard enough and exercise discipline, you can deserve to have all the things that make life worth living.[13] In the words of the brilliant fat activist, Virgie Tovar:

Diet culture does one thing very successfully: it alienates us from our natural relationship to food and movement, things that we as human beings have had a relationship to since the beginning of time, and which we cannot live without, and it sells them back to us as "diet" and "exercise" with the promise that with hard work and self-denial we can achieve a state worthy of love, respect and admiration.[14]

Like our confusion around happiness and property, we have another, fundamental misunderstanding about the relationship between food, eating, exercise, and our essential virtue. The trouble is they're *honestly not* related. The relationship is a fabrication.

The Sanctioned Language of Acceptable Femininity

Can you get through your day without seeing an image or hearing words that promote weight loss, either overtly or subliminally? To opt out of diet culture is an act of rebellion. To accept yourself and others as you and they are *now*—no matter what your looks—is a subversive act.

But for women, diet culture has created a concrete project for us to undertake to prove to the world that we are good and therefore deserving of all the wonderful things in life. Thinner = better.

It also creates socially sanctioned topics of obedient conversation:

- What did we eat yesterday?

- What we're planning to eat today.

- What we're going to do to get in shape for the summer.

- Oh, those danged holiday cookies are so evil and tempting, aren't they?

- It looks like Jane is "letting herself go," she's gained so much weight, it's such a tragedy.

- Judy has lost so much weight, she looks so great, I want to talk to her about what she's doing and how she did it; I'll tell you all about it.

- Do I look fat in this?

- I feel fat.

These topics, so common in women's relating to each other, diminish women's virtues, intelligence, and value. And the truly, *truly* sad part is, we do it to ourselves. No one forces us into these conversations. We perpetuate them. Therefore we also have an opportunity to *interrupt* them.

How?

- *What we ate yesterday?* becomes *what did I learn about yesterday?*

- *What we're planning to eat today* becomes *what pleasure I'm anticipating in this day.*

- *What we're going to do to get in shape this summer* becomes *what fun outdoor activity I'm looking forward to this summer.*

- *Those danged holiday cookies* becomes *all the fun I had making the holiday cookies.*

- *Jane's letting herself go* becomes *what's going on in Jane's life and how can we help?*

- *Judy lost so much weight* becomes *I wonder what's going on in Judy's life and whether she's well and happy?*

- *Do I look fat in this?* becomes *I'm feeling insecure about my appearance.*

- *I feel fat* becomes *something is bugging me; I can't quite put my finger on it.*

Refuse to take part in the conversation by skillfully and kindly redirecting. Set an example that upholds a vision of women's inherent human value.

Women's Bodies Are Naturally Good

Diet culture makes everything that is natural about a woman's body "bad."

Cellulite.

Jiggling.

Bouncing.

Curves.

Being soft to the eye and to the touch.

Back rolls.

Belly rolls.

Muffin tops.

Did I mention cellulite?

Diet culture takes all the wonderful, natural things about women's bodies and makes them "bad." Diet culture keeps women hating their bodies and therefore hijacks tremendous amounts of energy we might otherwise use to collectively ask more from the world. More for ourselves, and more on behalf of the good of the world.

Additionally, diet culture focuses women on an improvement project, which costs money. Spending money keeps capitalism churning. Money allows people to purchase property. Having property is the key to happiness (right?). And the glitch in this program is that happiness is *not* achieved through property. But since we've been trained that it is thus, we keep returning to this project and pumping more money into it.

It's a rather neat equation, if you think about it. The trouble is, this so-called happiness is built on the misery and self-hatred of half of our species—women. And this poisons the entire project at the root.

Our Bodies, Our Selves

Fundamentally, our culture, specifically diet culture, tells us as women that our bodies *are not our own.* Our bodies must be pleasing to others. If our bodies are not ours, then whose are they? Our Judeo-Christian culture gives this answer: your body belongs to God and to the church. And a female body has one real purpose: to reproduce.

The decision to claim your female body, completely and entirely for yourself—for your pleasure, for your enjoyment, for your definition of beauty, to reproduce or not, with whomever you want—is a truly modern and radical act. It shakes down *multiple generations* of ancestral inheritance. And it can both be radical *and* sacred, holding all the things you believe about your religion in place while simultaneously claiming and embodying spirit in every cell of your body.

Here's the truth. You can do what you want with your body. It's yours.

You can eat what you want.

You can wear what you want.

You can use it the way you want.

You can *change* it the way you want.

Hold it. How does "radical acceptance" make way for changing the body? Here's how: sometimes our bodies are not enough for us. We do all the internal work, and we just decide, *you know what? I really want a different nose. It's not about me hating my body, it's about me having a different vision of myself.* Sometimes you want what another has. Is it stupid or vain to get your breasts enlarged? Not necessarily. I think that arriving at the *why* of your rationale is an opportunity for personal growth, understanding, acceptance and transformation. I have a client who got herself some bigger breasts. And my stance was—I want you to be happy. It is your body. You are entitled to do with it—and *every part* of it—exactly what you want. I will love you regardless of what you look like, because *I value* you.

It's important that we, as women, never judge what another woman does with her body. If you believe that *your* body is yours, and you can do what you want with it, then we are duty-bound to preserve and protect that right for other women.

I believe this also holds true for people who have decided that they want to lose weight. Many of my family and friends are what society would call "overweight." Some of them are fine with that; others aren't. Some of them want to sign up with (what was once known of as) Weight Watchers and lose weight. By now you probably have gathered my stance on the losing weight project. Surrendering to diet culture? Maybe, maybe not. It depends on what is in your heart and mind when you make the decision. It's all in the intent.

But here's what I learned from a friend who studied with Marsha Linehan: you can't stop judging by judging judging. If my friends are judging themselves, my also judging them for that isn't going to stop the original judging. It's that simple. So what's the solution? Acceptance. Compassion. Understanding. In essence—love. These are the tools we need to have, and use, to cut through our culture of competition, comparison, judgment, and envy.

It's all in the intent.

THE GRASS LOOKS GREENER...WHERE?

My understanding of my friend Olivia was, for me, a journey which dissolved the energies of envy and judgment. Olivia is thin like most people long to be, the kind of thin that cameras and photographers love. Over the years of our friendship I discovered she struggled to maintain her weight, despite eating heartily. Olivia ate every high-calorie whole food she could get her hands on—peanut butter, butter, coconut oil. She would inadvertently lose weight if she didn't keep an eye on it. She regarded her body with disappointment because to her it wasn't "womanly" enough.

One Halloween, we planned to go out together, as it had become our annual tradition to attend a big dance party in New York. We got dressed and put on makeup at the yoga studio where we taught together and posed for pre-party photos. Olivia chose a Little Bo Peep costume, and I was a mermaid. Someone snapped Polaroids for us. Olivia peered at the photos with initial enthusiasm and then said, "Wow. You look like a woman. I look like a little girl." She was crestfallen.

Through comments like these I began to learn that she suffered in isolation over her appearance. As our friendship grew, I like to think and hope her suffering was less isolating and private, since she started to reveal to me more and more of her disparaging thoughts about her body.

I realized Olivia's silent suffering was compounded further by having a "desirable"—read *thin*—body. For the most part, she was unable to share her body confidence challenges without being seen as being ungrateful or narcissistic. Who wants to hear the skinny girl's complaints?

Nobody.

So she was forced further into isolation with her concerns. Knowing Olivia cracked open my mind and heart and started to change my thoughts (and envy!) about blonde, thin, attractive people, and by extension, *every person.*

A saying circulates in the yogi circles (and in social media memes), one that's a terrific antidote to envy: Be kind to everyone, for you can't know what battles people are fighting.

Everyone fights a battle we cannot imagine. We will *never know, never really understand.* Would you trade your problems for the unknown troubles of another person? Probably not!

Green Is the Color of Envy

When you compare your life to another's, find yours lacking, and want *what you think they have (but can't be sure your ideas are real or true),* this is envy.

The experience of envy involves:

- Feelings of inferiority

- Longing

- Resentment of circumstances

- Ill will toward the envied person, often accompanied by guilt about these feelings

- Motivation to improve

- Desire to possess the attractive rival's qualities

- Disapproval of feelings[15]

(A side note: people often conflate envy and jealousy. Envy is a reaction to lacking something. Jealously is a fear of losing something—usually a person—often to a third party.)

When I learned about Olivia's life and challenges, which diverged radically from what I imagined, my envy started to dissolve. As I realized that what I *thought* her experience was differed so vastly from her *reality*, I began to wonder about all the other people whose lives I envied. In what myriad of ways had I myself been cruel to them by assigning them emotional advantages that perhaps their exterior appearances didn't actually confer? As I considered these possibilities, and interacted with more "beautiful" people and from a place of genuine inquiry became curious about their lives and experiences, I began to know some of their very real body-related sorrows. As a result, my wounds of hurt, heartbreak, and self-doubt, which I had been carrying for so many years from that childhood experience with my blonde friends, began to heal.

Learning about other people's experience is the antidote to envy. When you find out about other people's lives and experiences, most often you will discover that what you envy in another comes with personal costs to them that you did not, maybe *could not*, perceive. The process of learning about other people widens your perception so that you can see and understand more. Understanding the costs of another person's experience builds empathy, and perhaps even compassion.

Understanding that having what they have will in fact *not* bring you any closer to the happiness you seek—this is a powerful and skillful move of critical awareness.

Learning about other people's experience is the antidote to envy.

For expert-level liberation, free yourself from your envy without even needing to know the suffering that accompanies another persons' circumstance. Everyone suffers. *That's all you need to know.* "Beautiful" people suffer. Rich people suffer. How and why? That's their own private story and mystery.

Envy Individuates

Envy can lead us to isolate or remove ourselves from the company of those who arouse the emotion. It can also cause us to individuate. Individuating is the act of thinking that *I am the only one*—with this brunette hair, or acne, or muffin-top problem, or—fill in the blank.

Self-consciousness and worrying about our weight keeps us trapped in ourselves. With my last weight gain of twenty pounds, I found myself individuating, thinking how I uniquely was suffering this horrible weight gain. I resented my body and resented life—*how dare my body do this! How unfair was life to make me experience this* again! I was certain that there was something wrong, as I couldn't exactly identify how it had happened. I felt uniquely punished by the universe. And finally, I felt ashamed of my belly and didn't want to reveal it. I thought that it was disgusting, and the fact that my stomach flesh touched my shirt was revolting and shameful. *Who would possibly go out of the house like this? How could any self-respecting person show herself like this?*

This thinking is toxic. And it's embarrassingly self-absorbed. Look at the preceding paragraph. How many "I's" are there? When you see writing or hear speech like this, it tells you that people are really wrapped up in themselves and their own experiences. They are individuating.

Thinking only about yourself shuts out empathy and compassion—for other people *and,* interestingly, for yourself. Heart energy makes a wonderful, self-nourishing loop. When you feel for others, it helps you to feel compassion for your own struggles. For me, teaching is a powerful tool to get out of my own head, because I am working in service of others.

Hearing others' stories about their challenges can aid us too, which is one reason why body-image memoirs are very healing. They help us realize that *we are not alone.* There are other people who are suffering and struggling in a similar way, and simply knowing this can ease our burden. Feeling alone, isolated, and individuated is often a significant part of our suffering. This is why I created my Adore Your Body Telesummit and interviewed colleagues and friends about *their* body-image challenges—to help other women realize that *they are not alone!* (See the Resource Guide at the end of the book.)

> *If you're having a difficult day, doing something of service for another is a good way to pull yourself out of it.*

Advice for Disrupting Sanctioned Feminine Conversations

I want to preface what I'm about to explain by saying: I *want* you to opt out of diet culture. I want you to disavow it forever. (Opting out of diet culture opens the door for you to explore caring for your body though self-determined constructive food choices and pleasurable movement.) But, weirdly, diet culture also includes opportunities to connect with other people. While I certainly *don't* recommend building relationships and connections on strengthening the bonds of diet culture—which is often what women do when they talk about their diets and exercise—one very small consolation prize is that it opens the door for people to discuss their experience. Asking "Do I look fat in this?"—self-defeating though it may be—is an opportunity for the people involved in that heartbreaking inquiry to break down the walls of isolation and talk to others. We might view it as a call for help. And we, as fiercely aware women, can hear the common female points of connection (about food, diet, exercise, clothes) as opportunities to go deeper into a more poignant, honest conversation about ourselves, our longings, and our heartbreaks. Here are healthy new ways to connect, steeped in compassion and curiosity.

- *When someone starts talking about what they are going to eat,* ask them how it makes them feel to eat in a certain way, and why they have made that decision.

- *When someone starts talking about "bad" food,* ask them why it's bad, and how they arrived at that decision, and what they feel they have accomplished by not eating it.

- *When someone starts talking about their exercise regimen,* ask them where they learned it, and why they do it, and how it makes them feel, and how it empowers them in their lives.

- *When someone starts talking about how "bad" someone else looks* (they've gained weight, they've "let themselves go," they look run down), take the opportunity to muse about what might be happening for that person and to generate compassion for the circumstances of their lives.

- *When someone starts talking about how "good" someone else looks* because they've lost weight, take the opportunity to talk about what might be happening in their lives to create those circumstances. Sometimes people lose weight when they are happy. Others lose weight when they are under enormous stress, or have experienced heartbreak, or even when they are sick—or *dying!*

That dumb old diet culture creates predictable conversations we can disrupt. We can plan for them, considering how we want to respond in new, expansive ways. Contemplate all the spaces where people *don't* have an opportunity to talk about their experience. For instance, how do thin people who feel bad about their bodies open this door to discussion? Recall my friend Olivia—there is no cultural norm for her. In fact, I think that even thin people absorb the message that the only way to discuss their discomfort is to talk about "feeling fat." Have you ever had someone who is truly, truly thin say to you "I feel fat"? This way of expressing ourselves has become a compulsion and its own pathology, because we've lost the ability to identify, understand, and express what is *really* bothering us. What we're saying when we say "I feel fat" is some version of "There's something wrong with me" or "I'm having an uncomfortable emotion that I can't quite identify, so I'll reach for my default, a problem I can solve: *I feel fat.*" Then you might mistakenly think you can solve "the problem" by losing weight or otherwise seeking to modify your body. It doesn't work.

"Feeling fat" becomes a proxy for all kinds of other anxieties about ourselves:

- Our lovability

- Our worthiness

- Our desirability

- Feelings of loneliness

- Abandonment

- An absence of experiencing respect

And this is just to name a few particularly gnarly emotional quagmires.

If we can identify this tendency, then when one of our friends says to us, "I feel fat" we can help and support and guide her to understand the *real* underlying emotion and then deal with it on its own terms. You might inquire, "Babe, what's that *really* about?"

So often we are left alone to suffer and try to make sense of our bodily experience. In isolation, people are far more likely to arrive at far-fetched conclusions, like *There's something wrong with me.* This thought breeds shame and creates a loop that reinforces a painful cycle.

Critical awareness of our personal experience, how we relate in our society, and how life works, is key to our undoing the cycle of envy, shame, and suffering around our bodies. Understand this: the grass is *never* greener. People are battling their own personal demons. Fat people suffer. Thin people suffer. Having a body is a real challenge! Recognizing this fundamental truth builds compassion and dissipates envy. When those dark emotions disappear, it's healing for those on the receiving end; meanwhile, producing and experiencing noble emotions (compassion, understanding) from within also heals us. You are healing yourself by generating noble emotions! This is good medicine for all involved, and you are on the path to creating that in the world. How beautiful!

What to Do When Others Envy You

Envy harms the person who feels it. But it also hurts the person who is its target. It's poisonous for both parties.

The influential Danish philosopher, Søren Kierkegaard, believed that there are types of people who arouse envy and are as guilty when it arises as those who feel it. And some people take pleasure in making others feel inferior. Envy is often a problem for those of great natural beauty or talent.

On the subject of receiving envy, Robert Greene, author of *The 48 Laws of Power*, suggests first of all acquiring the self-awareness to understand that you might inspire envy in others. Without awareness of your own effect on other people, you will be helpless to do anything.

I developed early. Any clinical psychologist will tell you that "early developers" are exponentially more prone to low self-esteem than late developers, and this proved true for me.

Even on the edge of puberty I was already tall, and in fifth grade I towered above my teacher. My peers did what children often do to anomalies—they ridiculed me. A sensitive child, already attuned to the ways that children hurt one another, I was deeply affected and internalized the message that I was weird and unattractive. It was only once I moved to New York City, at twenty-nine, that I began to understand I was neither. Men of all ages and ethnicities seemed to think my tall, busty, brunette looks were mighty fine, thank you! I had a fundamental misperception about my appearance and its impact on others.

New York men were approving. Women were another matter.

One year, celebrating Olivia's birthday, a group had drinks at a swim-up bar in New York. It was girls-only, and we all came with our bikinis. Eyeing me critically, one gal quipped, "Nice knockers, Erica." I immediately felt ashamed, like maybe I looked bad in my bikini, or maybe my breasts were displayed in some immodest way—oh my, where did this flood of shame come from?

As we all know, our society tells us breasts are especially attractive when they're big. Because I was an early developer, boys and girls alike made fun of my breasts in middle school. In what I believe was my parents' effort to protect me from people who might mistake their fourteen-year-old daughter for a twenty-one-year-old, they always encouraged me to *cover up!* In the context of my poor self-esteem and body image, I could hardly understand why girls were so mean to me about my breasts. I thought that they must be really ugly. The mixed messages were confusing and made me feel crazy.

You can probably see, in light of this history, how the incident at the swim-up bar was upsetting. The next day I wept in the arms of one of my male yoga-teaching buddies, Joseph. He patted my back, and smoothed my hair and said, "Don't mind them, love. They're just jealous." (He misused the word—he really meant envious, but at the time I didn't understand the distinction. Nevertheless, I got his gist.)

I couldn't compute what he was saying. Jealous? Of me? Whatever for?

And then, for some reason, that day it started to sink in. *I don't look like what I think I look like. Ohhhhh…*

As I slowly came to understand that I wasn't really oafish and ugly like I had imagined, I had two heartbreaking epiphanies about myself and the effect I have on other people.

1. I inadvertently make some women feel bad about themselves.

2. Some women try to shame me about my body in order to make themselves feel better about *their* feelings of envy, guilt, and shame (this is a common strategy people use to handle their own feelings of envy).

Holy smokes! All these years, was the mirror lying to me about the way I look, or was I just *not able to see what is real?* I began to understand that my *mind* was the thing to question. Not the mirror. The mirror is simply an inanimate object. My mind interprets what it sees.

In the face of these epiphanies, my perception widened and my heart also expanded, *because I understood the suffering of the people who aimed to hurt me.* Suddenly I felt connected to all the women who had felt envious of another woman.

Thanks to receiving this convoluted, painful education about how our bodies shape our experiences, I was reminded how our interior experience rarely matches our exterior circumstances. How apt the expression, *never judge a book by its cover.*

Understanding how you might arouse other people's envy, and their coping mechanisms, can grow your heart, help you to become a more compassionate person, and prepare you to respond with grace.

We are at a very important moment in history for women. We have an opportunity to celebrate one another and lift each other up as we never have before. Envy has divided us. We must dissolve it.

How?

Simple: a hearty dose of admiration for one another.

First, recognize what kinds of environments are conducive to envy, among colleagues, peers, and even close friends. The two greatest tools I've acquired are offering another sincere praise and working to lift others up. Women are taught to hide their skills and to be self-deprecating, so these tools can be very beneficial. When you feel envy arising around you in the form of comparison, competition, or judgment, recognize that your talents and assets may be on display in a way that others feel uncomfortable exhibiting themselves. It may not simply be that you are amazing (which you are), but also that you feel comfortable being *seen for the truth of who and what you are*. That variety of safe feeling, which some might describe as confidence, may be something others long for and therefore envy.

I want women to thrive together, without hiding. Therefore we must become great admirers of others' successes. It's certainly one fine way to appreciate all of the beauty in the world. Here's what you can do: select a girlfriend to brag with. Yes, brag! In these brag sessions, talk openly about all the great things that you've accomplished. Squeal! Applaud! Decide how and when you're going to celebrate! Make this a common feature of your female friendships. Become generous in your appreciation for the good fortune of the people around you. This energy is good for them and also good medicine for you.

Envy is a certain kind of emotional weather. Notice that you are experiencing it. Accept all that you feel while also resisting the urge to objectify the person of whom you feel envious, to compare, or to judge. Resist the urges to *allow* your thinking to move you toward shame, resentment, or hatred. Make an effort to get to know about that person's unique experience. As you do so, you will make them human and start to know about their particular form of suffering. From there you might begin to empathize with them. You may even find you prefer *your* personal challenges to theirs. This will transform you *and* the people around you! Reframed this way, I hope you see envy as a wonderful opportunity.

GREEN IS THE COLOR OF THE HEART CHAKRA

Every day we have a choice. We can let the events of our lives harden our hearts. We can go through our lives angry, and sad, and bitter. Or we can use the difficult events of our lives to wake up, and practice conditioning our hearts to be strong and resilient, and flexible and courageous.

Envy is an energy that closes and hardens the heart. Can you feel that? It's an energy that makes us the victim in our own story, instead of the hero.

In so many contemplative philosophies, the thing that heals all is some version of heart energy. Love. Compassion. Forgiveness. It shows up as the central tenet of Christianity, Buddhism, and yoga too. I'm just tickled how the color green, the color associated with envy, is also connected with the heart chakra, in the chakra system.

Chakra translates as "wheel," and the chakras are considered part of the "subtle body." The chakras are seven energy points, each corresponding with a nerve plexus, that runs the length of the spine and into the skull. They are hubs of energetic activity in both the physical and metaphysical bodies. They're like a radio tower that plugs us into the ground and extends us into the sky.

You can explore the complete chakra system more on your own to expand your understanding of your own body in a mystical way. For our purposes here, we'll focus on the relevant chakra.

In every explanation of the chakras, the fourth is always in relationship to love, because it corresponds with the anatomical heart. In fact, often it's just called "the heart chakra."

Ana Forrest identifies the main issue of the fourth chakra as the quest of the Warrior's Heart. What does it mean to quest for and have a warrior's heart? Essentially it means that we battle with our own dragons. Our dragons are our triggers, our ugly emotions, and our damaging behaviors. The warrior's heart is our willingness to use the events of our lives to help us hunt down and flush out our fears and become fearless. It's our unwavering commitment to using our life challenges to grow our own heart's capacity for holding the messy contradictions that come with being human, and thereby to feel more, to break wide open, and to grow bigger and bigger inside. Ultimately our quest for a warrior's heart brings us always nearer to clarity of heart. When we allow the events of our lives to harden us, this also obscures our ability to perceive what is real and true. You may be familiar with this quote from Antoine De Saint-Exuprey's timeless classic *The Little Prince:* "It is only with the heart that one can see rightly; what is essential is invisible to the eye."

A true yogi is one who is *fearless* and has *purity of heart.* Heart practices that I've learned, discovered, and practiced in my yoga are part of the way that we clean up the heart, dismantle its armor, and open it. Purity of heart means that we dissolve our resistance to the truth.

Our heart functions with its own intelligence. It has its own language, one that we risk forgetting if we stop keeping our heart healthy and listening to it. In *The Alchemist,* Paulo Coelho warns us that when we stop listening to our heart, it stops communicating.[16] We must not underestimate the wisdom of this insight. Our bodies possess their own intelligences, and within each body are smaller components and systems, like the heart, with their own unique intelligence. Our society is functioning on a shortfall of the energies that the heart produces and provides—compassion, love, forgiveness—and this harms us as individuals and as a whole. The deficit breaks our hearts, makes them weak and susceptible to diseases and emotional distress. Helping our hearts be strong, resilient, and healthy will help us counter our tendencies toward comparison, judgment, and envy.

An Exercise to Take Care of Your Heart

A universal symbol of the heart's energies is a rose, and the colors of the heart chakra are green and pink, like the stem and blossom of a pink rose. For all of you who vibe on symbolism and visualization, can you feel the vibration of those two colors in your heart space? Take that image into this embodied exercise.

Put your hands over your chest. Feel the warmth of your hands against your chest. Inhale, and feel the expansion of your lungs and the lift of your ribs. Grow your breath on the front of your heart. Take three to five more breaths, expanding your breath capacity there. When you exhale, maintain the lift in your spine and ribs, pulling your low belly back toward your spine. If you are a visualizer, see your favorite flower growing from the front of your heart.

Now move your hands to the sides of your ribcage. Feel the pressure of your hands on your ribs. Inhale and expand your ribs outward against your hands. Feel this expansion. This is "side of heart" territory. When you breathe in, pay attention to the sensation of your breath as it swells the side of your heart. How does it feel? Take three to five more breaths, working to grow your breath capacity there. When you exhale, maintain the lift in your spine and ribcage, pulling your low belly back toward your spine to help. If you are a visualizer, see your favorite flower growing from your side ribs.

Now move your hands to your back, or lie down to feel the back of the heart connection to the floor. Inhale and expand your back ribs. This is "back of heart" territory. Grow your breath into the back of your heart, focusing on expanding your back ribs with each inhale. Take three to five more breaths into this region, paying attention to the physical sensations, and potentially to the emotional sensations that arise. How does it feel? If you are a visualizer, see your favorite flower growing from your back. You are a flower.

Now choose one of these three areas to repeat. Make your choice based on a first flash of curiosity, need, or desire. Go back to that heart territory and give it three or five more deep breaths, growing your breath capacity there, and feeling for the sensations of your heart.

This is a good, simple way to begin creating a bodily, feeling-based relationship with your heart. Do it daily. And then begin to also ask of your heart "What do you want today?" Begin a daily "heart log," noting what it asks for. As you are able, do your best to satisfy those heartfelt desires.

The heart is part of the physical body. It's an organ. And it also is an energy center, a feature of your subtle body. Many of us have never been taught how to take care of this aspect of our heart, and when this is missing, our self-hatred can *break our own heart*. We are not meant to hate ourselves! We are meant to *love* ourselves.

Hating ourselves leads to more heartbreak, and not of the good, opening-up variety. It's the kind of heartbreak that leads us to want to shut down, close up shop, and armor ourselves forever. What we *need*, desperately, is to open our hearts—to ourselves, to our bodies, to others who also need to open their hearts to their bodies. Loving your body is at the core of this radical body acceptance project. Learning to love, to have compassion for your body, must be, by definition, an *embodied experience!* These are *embodied* practices, so they *must* involve your body, as both the subject and the recipient of the energies involved.

When we experience envy, we look at our neighbor's grass and think it's greener. When we experience compassion, we feel for our neighbors; we lean over the fence and offer to help them to plant roses.

Let's check in. How are you feeling? How is your *body* responding to everything that you're learning? In the prior lesson, I mentioned that absorbing this information is an organic process that takes time, like digestion of food (relatively fast), or a garden growing (slower, over many years). Feel in right now for what would help you with this organic digestion and growth process. A nap? A walk? A conversation with a friend? What do you need? How can you give it to yourself?

Envy denies us our true longings and desires.

Perhaps you're feeling quite overwhelmed and not actually able to recall the contents of the lesson. It might be helpful to know this can be the body's strategy for dealing with stress and overwhelm—short-term memory loss. It's as if whatever was just upsetting didn't happen! Neat trick, right?

The learning in this "The Grass Is *Never* Greener" chapter may take a while for you to absorb, or it may take root overnight. So much of what our culture teaches us regarding comparison and competition is unnatural that you might find yourself so enchanted by *how good it feels* to admire the people around you that you never want to compare, compete, or judge ever again.

Here's the truth. What your face and body look like is predominantly the result of divine inspiration, a creative force that makes no mistakes. You, darling, are a work of art! This art might not be to your taste, but as my teacher Alison Armstrong says, "You did not paint your face." It's out of your hands (unless you have a lot of money and a talented plastic surgeon!). Doing battle with these things is a waste of energy. Consider yourself a steward and a curator of the art that is your body and your face. Take care of yours! Evaluating yours compared to others' is also a big waste of time. Admire yours and everyone else's! Try it. You will find out that being an aficionada of people and their unique beauty feels so good that you may never ever want to go back into the space of comparison, judgment, competition, or envy. Teaching yoga taught me to admire humanity. People are very mysterious, and very beautiful. All of them.

And if you find yourself still pulled into the weeds, judging, comparing, competing, well, then, I advise you revisit the "Staying Unhappy" section in Lesson 1 and *go deeper!* Some gardens simply need more attention than others. With enough, your own grass will look mighty verdant to you, indeed.

Turn Poison into Good Medicine

As a child athlete and swimmer I became aware of a discrepancy between what I saw in the media and in "real life." I observed bodies, played the comparison game, and noticed how the human form is *infinitely varied.* As a matter of fact, no one on the swim team had a body even remotely resembling the underwear models in Victoria's Secret. There's a huge incongruity between what the media portrays as ideal and the way people really are. We're fed fantasy.

Observing bodies, it dawned on me that "perfect" is a fixed, immobile point, like the center of a bull's-eye. Rockettes and Victoria's Secret models are hired for their uniformity and proximity to that fixed point. But for "perfect" to truly exist, each and every person would need to agree that whatever "it" is—legs, butts, noses—is perfect. All of us would have to agree—*yes, that is perfect!* It's impossible to get everyone everywhere to agree; therefore, logically, perfect does not, *cannot* exist.

I drew these conclusions:

- No one I knew looked like anyone in those magazines.

- Everybody's body was utterly distinct.

- A "perfect" body does not exist.

If you look around, you too will notice that the bodies identified as "beautiful" are also rare. In fact, less than 4 percent of the population have fashion-model dimensions. Scarcity generates value. But here's an alternative view: if some greater power meant for us to look just one way, then why does everyone look so *different?* If that uniformity were considered valuable, special, and blessed, then why are there 8.7 *million* distinct species on the earth? If a thigh gap were preferred, then how come most women's thighs rub together? Human values are small inventions of a small mind. The one force that created this universe finds value in the vastness of variety.

What if our thighs are *meant* to rub together? Meditate on that, and think about your thighs rubbing together when you walk, and *move* like this is right, amazing, and…divine. Find out what happens!

Difference is meant not to divide us, but to bring us together.

The divine is found in diversity. The force that created you does not make mistakes. Your value resides in your uniqueness. When *through* our differences we *arrive* at unity, this is enlightened existence.

THE VALUE EQUATION OF A BODY: LOOKS, DOES, FEELS

Disliking how the body *looks,* we'll often redefine its value equation in new terms, primarily *what it can do,* and *what it does for me.* These are good and useful steps in rehabilitating your relationship with your body, but I find that too often it's a way in which we deny how we *really* feel about our looks. Truthfulness is the only way toward transformation, so it's imperative to be honest about our feelings.

Like many others do on this journey, I began to focus on what my body could *do,* and my obsession with exercise increased. *If my body is not beautiful or thin, at least it can be useful and strong.*

After high school, I joined my collegiate crew team. Rowing fed my masochistic urge to test my body's limits. After a year, I burned out and left the team, but continued to work out, a minimum of two hours a day, seven days a week. I became a compulsive over-exerciser. I thought I was achieving two virtuous goals:

- Exercise to be thin

- Exercise to be strong

I'm a strong and capable athlete; there was no doubt my body could *do* things. The problem was, I still hated myself. Built on self-loathing, this exercise compulsion was completely unsustainable energetically, physically, financially, and emotionally. Pursuits founded on fear, hate, or lies will eventually crumble. Operate from love, joy, and trust.

See, you can't hate yourself into loving yourself, yet that's what so many of us are doing. When you exercise while hating yourself, you bathe the body in poisonous thoughts and turn your internal pharmacopeia into a toxic cesspool. It's only a matter of time before something gives.

My new value equation—the body is valuable for what it can *do,* for how strong, fast, or capable I am—just wasn't working out.

When you notice yourself valuing your body exclusively for its ability to do things, follow these steps.

1. Recognize it. It's okay! It's a step moving along the path from valuing the body for what it looks like to valuing what it *is.* It's part of a self-valuing system that you *want to have.* It just can't be the only factor.

2. Consider: if you were unable to continue to do those things, where might you source your self-value from?

3. What do you think it would feel like to just appreciate your body for existing? Think of someone you love just...because you *do.* This can be a "feeling map" for you to identify how you could one day feel about yourself.

Pursuits founded on fear, hate, or lies will eventually crumble. Operate from love, joy, and trust.

ADDICTED TO PERFECTION

There are certain compulsions we readily accept because they're "healthy" behaviors. Here are the top three:

- Work

- Exercise

- Diet

We attach virtue to these endeavors. In our pursuit of perfection, we overlook the dark side of "getting it right."

When I was an exercise addict, my days were dominated by the need to move. Just like any addict, I was savage until I got my fix. At the time, I didn't see the exercise for what it was—self-abuse. I was on a quest for an improved version of myself, and I experienced relief from emotional pain only while momentarily making myself "better." When not exercising and not actively involved in that pursuit, the pain of "not improving right now" would become overwhelming. And if I didn't exercise, I was "bad."

Many of us conceal our self-loathing behind "acceptable" addictions, like exercise, work, or diet.

The paradox is, in moderate doses, work, healthy food, and exercise are good ideas. They're things you *need* to do! What's tricky is when the very things we must do daily—especially eating and working—become bad for us. Everything in moderation. Even the good stuff.

Everything in moderation. Even the good stuff.

I believe that humans are inherently addictive creatures. It's nothing personal, simply a foible of the species. We seek to self-soothe through habits, routines, excitement, or risk. We'll need these things to feel... something. These attachments are okay until they start to run us.

Let's find out what you're hooked on. Get out your journal and title a new page "What Kind of Perfection Addict Am I?"

1. Can you identify if you have an "activity addiction" that's truly a cover-up for pursuing perfection? Feel within for something that you feel has to be "just so" or you don't feel grounded or simply aren't the person you recognize as yourself. The slippery challenge is that our routines (morning coffee, a walk) truthfully make us feel "better" but without them we are a worse version of ourselves. The uplevel is to *still* strive to be the best version of yourself even in the absence of your routines.

2. When you identify your "acceptable addiction," feel in to find out what pain you are working to avoid. You might not be able to identify what that pain is, yet. Continue to quest after the answer. Often we'll build up our personalities in defense against the parts of ourselves we disapprove of most.

    •   If you work too much—find out how you would fill your time if you didn't. If you stop working and discover that you feel panicked, take a few breaths and stay with the feeling before you launch yourself into a new project. Inquire into how you would like to spend your life besides working. What experiences would you like to have? Write those down. If they're only "big" things like going to Machu Picchu, find out what little "daily" experiences you'd like to have more of. Begin to fill your extra time with those delights.

    •   If you exercise too much—identify activities that engage your body in movement that is only for the pleasure of it. There's no outcome expected, no achievement. Simply the enjoyment of movement. List three, at least. Five, for more freedom.

    •   If you eat too much, or worry about food too much, or eat too little—find out what feelings you are trying to soothe. Anxious, and trying to ground yourself? What are some other methods you could also try? Lonely, and filling up that void? Starving to become invincible? Reach out, and fill up your life with more human connection or even animal connection. Lacking sweetness in your life, so you fill up on sugary foods? Find out what your heart and your spirit are craving in the form of sweetness in your life.

3. You might have an addiction that *isn't* socially approved. The steps here similar. What pain are you seeking to soothe, and what are you avoiding? Start to address these realities on their own terms.

4. Finally, get support! Buddy up! It's helpful to have people who are working on the same changes to go through it together. Who do you think you could rely on in this area? List them.

It might be surprising to discover your acceptable addiction, and this revelation might produce other, confronting emotions—such as shame, anger, resistance. You might feel angry *with me* for pointing it out! These are all okay and natural. Remember that the first step is to acknowledge the truth and reality of these emotions. You're getting stronger all the time, and you can handle yourself!

GOING COLD TURKEY ON POISONOUS PERFECTION

The breaking point in my exercise addiction came in the form of a message from on high. One day my wiser self whispered to the insane over-exerciser: "You cannot hate yourself into loving yourself."

I didn't *want* to go on hating myself; this wasn't the person I envisioned myself to be! Moreover, there was no light on the horizon—if I continued this way, I could anticipate spending the rest of my life at the gym, hating myself for not looking perfect. *If you want to see your future, look at what you are doing today.* Based on what I was doing day to day, I had a clear picture of my future.

> You cannot hate yourself into loving yourself.

Presented with this dim view of the path ahead, overnight I stopped exercising. I sat on my butt for about two years, doing nothing even faintly resembling exercising. I couldn't trust myself to not get hooked again. Removing the outward expression of my self-loathing exposed its roots, and I began weeding my garden of dark thoughts. My exhaustion and heartbreak came into clear view. Hating yourself is *tiring*!

Addictions are hard to give up. Compulsions are hard to let go of. But love and compulsion cannot coexist.

If we agree to loosen our grip, or to take away the things standing between us and our sadness, we must come face to face with our most troubling inner shadows and the most unsettling questions about our lives. The truth is, sometimes our addictions just seem easier than the work we're confronted with when our "drug" of choice is removed.

We're antagonized by questions like these:

- Why do I dislike myself so much?

- Will I ever feel better?

- How can I get what I want?

- How can I feel better about myself?

Love and compulsion cannot coexist.

- Will I ever have the life that I think I want?

- What am I here for?

- What am I doing with my life?

- How can I get the things that I need and want from life and the people around me?

In *so* many ways, numbing out using drugs or an acceptable addiction might seem like a better and easier path than dealing with these difficult questions.

Perfectionism is a poisoned apple. It seems righteously tasty at first, but eating it slowly kills your spirit.

The good news is, you can turn the poison into good medicine. Our greatest vulnerabilities are also our greatest opportunities for growth. When you recognize what difficult emotion is actually running you, you have a chance to become an honestly brighter, more brilliant version of yourself.

Ask yourself, is there just one compulsive behavior that you can commit to stopping today? It can be a small one. A way of thinking is a behavior. You might start with some of your internal attitudes, like disinterest or detachment. Envy, comparison, competing, and judging can be powerful habits to give up! You might begin with the way you speak—like gossiping, or complaining, or self-denigration. Go on a cleanse, like ninety days with no complaining, and find out what happens. Or there might be an outward action you're prepared to give up; say, for the next week, don't bring your smartphone with you when you [fill in your challenge: go to the gym, go to the bathroom, go for a hike...]Where will you begin?

Whenever you stop doing something, you've created a vacuum where that thought, speech, or behavior used to be. You might just want to experience the space for a while. Or you might need to fill it immediately. Whatever you do, be sure that you fill that space with thoughts, speech, or behavior steeped in kindness, compassion, generosity, and serenity.

Wherever you begin, you have taken the first small step toward something tremendous. Congratulations!

MIRROR, MIRROR ON THE WALL

Perfection has a leading role in the history of our relationship to feminine beauty. Our habits of judgment and comparison require something external to evaluate ourselves *against*. Looking in the mirror tells us what we look like. Visual representations of others supply objects of comparison. And there's an even more rarefied, etheric, universal ideal—a standard of beauty.

Small changes lead to big ones.

Are you aware of the standard to which you hold yourself? Within us we all have an idea of ourselves and how we measure up, as compared to the perfect or ideal woman. *But who is she? Where did she come from?*

From a historical perspective, women first inherited a sense of the ideal feminine through monotheistic religion. We were trained how to behave as compared to God, because God is perfect, God is love, and God is also beautiful.

God = Perfection

God = Love

God = Beauty

———————————————————————

Perfection = Love = Beauty

Visual representations of God depicted in art have also shaped our sense of perfection. The logic is:

God = Perfect

God = Good

———————————————————————

Perfect = Good

If: Perfection = Beauty = Love

And: Perfect = Good

———————————————————————

Good = Beauty

Perfection is portrayed as beautiful.

Therefore, to be beautiful is also to be good.

Perfection is good, and beautiful, and lovable.

This is how we often make the mistake of assuming that physically attractive people are also good or lovable.

Kings and queens staked *their* claim on perfectionism because they were the *human incarnations of God.* Their likenesses survived because they were painted. As visual media has become increasingly ubiquitous, new kinds of people have become "gods." It used to be that the "beautiful ones" were celebrities, actors, and entertainers. Now a person need not even possess a talent or skill to make it into the public eye. Beauty and good photos will suffice.

Advertising also affects people's ideas of perfection. Historically, models have tended to be pretty uniform in design. (Though these days we're entering a new era of diversity in representation!) Advertising tells us there's a wonderful land somewhere where perfect ladies lounge on beaches in bikinis or run buoyantly through tall grass, smiling like they have not a care in the world, because *beauty* earns a person a life of leisure. *Just buy this product and you will experience all of this too!* Advertising also suggests to us that "goodness," economic blessings, and leisure go hand in hand.

Since only 4 percent of people possess the precise genetics for classic model proportions, the beauty ideal is simply out of reach for almost all of us. But because of the moral equations I outlined earlier, perfectionism demands that we try anyway—otherwise we've abandoned all effort toward the virtue bound up in "trying," and therefore we are not *good*.

This is an (extremely) abbreviated history of the moral values packed into our beauty ideals. It's complex and twisted. Just to further confuse, it can even be used deceptively, as when great evil is portrayed as beautiful. Like the queen in *Snow White!* Just remember that you didn't invent any of this! You were born into a world where these constructs were already in place. To master them and to master yourself, it helps to understand the constructs. *Once you understand the rules, then you can break them.*

What steps can you take to help yourself? Here are a few:

1. To disrupt the power that visual representations of beauty have on us, cleanse your visual space of reinforcing depictions. You have a considerable amount of control over what you see daily. Take the reins. Television, magazines, and social media feeds are important places to begin. Cancel magazine subscriptions that portray women in ways that degrade your mood. Unfollow social media accounts that make you feel bad about yourself. Follow people who widen your perception of what is beautiful. Take note of what this

does for your brain, and see if you actually have become addicted to consuming harmful images, or even addicted to the process of "improving" yourself or comparing yourself to the images that you can see.

2. Consider what you think your own perfect woman looks like, how she acts, and how she behaves. If you were ever to measure up, what do you think you would get in return? When you ponder further, are you very certain that your return on investment will materialize? If you become unsure of the outcome, how might you spend your time and energy instead?

3. Start to orient your aspirations for being a better version of yourself toward a generous rendition. The hallmark of per-fectionism is that its qualities are contracting. There's scar-city. Your higher self is a better version of you, in which all of the emotions and experiences around you are limitless: joy, generosity, and kindness. These attributes are expansive, and they improve you *and* the people around you. There's abundance.

4. Finally, consider that, collectively, humans have misinter-preted the notion of "perfection" and its relationship with the divine. It's not that we must aspire to be "like God" but that God makes no mistakes, and as such *you* are perfect just the way you are.

It's natural to want to improve yourself; this is the path of an evolving soul. The error is in seeking improvement through a human notion of perfection, which takes us down the wrong path, the path of scarcity. A human mind thinks there can only be *one* person who is the fairest of them all! This mind-set denies the vast and varied beauty of the world and blinds us to all of the splendor existing around us *right now!* You have an opportunity right now to course-correct. This is very exciting!

PERFECTIONISM WASTES PRECIOUS HUMAN CAPITAL

Perfectionism would have us spend ourselves into a bottomless pit of diminishing returns. I fervently believe the future of our species hinges on body confidence and embodiment. (*Embodiment,* as I'll detail later, means integrating all the aspects of yourself in your body and fully experiencing the feelings of living from within your body.) The perfection project is so poisonous it threatens our very survival! It's a question of world peace and of human value, labor, and economics. I'll explain.

What currencies do you trade in? Here are some examples: there's emotional labor, intellectual labor, physical labor, spiritual labor. And all of them *cost* you something: *energy.*

We all have the same finite currencies:

- Money

- Energy

- Time

Spending time hating your body or pursuing a delusion of perfection *costs* you. It's time that you could spend in so many other ways, but once gone, you'll never get it back. You'll *never* recoup your investment price.

It also costs *energy.* The emotional toll of self-loathing is high. It's exhausting! You're probably also losing *money* in some way, shape, or form that you have not otherwise observed or tallied. Perfectionism drains away our personal currencies, throwing our energetic economics into deficit.

If you were to spend the time and energy caught up in hating your body in other ways, how would you spend it, and on what, and where in your life?

This is one of the central questions of this book and of life, and *the* essential point of our journey together. We're often unsure of how to spend our personal capital, so we dither it away daily on activities that amount to little or nothing over the long haul.

Sometimes the wasteful habits arise from a self-defeating loop. If we don't know what we want to do with our one precious life, then the time and energy spent on body concerns doesn't seem like time wasted. But there's a problem built in here: to discover how we want to spend our life, we might need to free up time and energy, which means spending less time and energy elsewhere.

For example, once, in my work life, I found myself spending far too much time commuting. I wanted that time back. I wasn't sure for what; I just knew that I wanted it back.

So I moved closer to work, freeing up time. Then I didn't know what to do with it. Uncertainty made me uncomfortable. So I filled the space with more work—and probably a lot of emotional eating to deal with discomfort.

This is an example of poor "human economics." It's a microcosm of how each person handles and spends their limited capital of time and energy. Self-loathing thoughts are an example of "leaking resources," because negative thoughts drain our time and energy. It's exhausting and stressful to think bad thoughts about ourselves! Overworking because we don't know what to do otherwise is another example of leaking resources. It might seem worthwhile, because work produces money, but unless you have a clear destination, you're spinning your wheels and might end up realizing you've wasted finite time.

Our time and energy are limited resources. Concern yourself with spending them in ways that raise your personal capital. If someone said to you, "Hey, do you want to waste 15 percent of your money today?" you would say "Hell no!" *But this is what we do with our time and energy!* Yikes! Consider for a moment what percentage of your time you spend in body dissatisfaction, and the emotional toll it takes. Honestly—put a number on it! Then assess how much it *costs* you. Write it in your journal now! Title this investigation, "What My Perfectionism Costs Me."

Time = ?

Price Tag = ?

If we all spent our precious time and energy hating ourselves *even 10 percent less* it would collectively elevate our human potential astronomically. Just imagine what we might do with ourselves, if we had just 10 percent more confidence, determination, and direction in our lives. What would it do to collective productivity? Would the GDP go up more than 3 percent? 10 percent? *What would it do, for you, in your life? How would it affect the people around you—your friends, your family, and your loved ones?* These are not rhetorical questions: really consider this! Take the time to journal on these questions!

You are not here to pour your life force down the drain into the perfection project or to spend your precious money on it.

The final currency of our human economics is money. Each year, our quest for perfection in the US feeds a $38 billion hair industry, a $33 billion diet industry, a $24 billion skincare industry, a $18 billion makeup industry, a $15 billion perfume industry, and a $13 billion cosmetic surgery industry.[17] This is a lot of money! I'm not suggesting you forgo grooming yourself, or that fashion and beauty aren't *fun*—I'm just pointing out that it's possible we're overspending money in areas that actually don't provide the return on investment we believe it promises!

Stop this madness! Let's divert more of our precious human capital of time, energy, and money to efforts that are real, compassionate, and will make a difference in the world. When we stop secretly hating ourselves, this creates a huge ripple effect in the collective psyche. When we free up *all* our currencies—time, money, energy—from wasteful habits, we restore our collective strength and prepare for a breakthrough.

You've already understood a critical truth by investing in perfectionism: *you* are your product. But instead of investing it materialism and externalities, why not spend your finite resources on education and experiences? These are real investments in becoming your wiser self.

You are not here to pay your bills.

What kinds of experiences do you want to have in your life? Who do you want to be? Invest in *becoming*.

HOW PERFECTIONISM POISONS (AND SLOWLY KILLS) US

Perfectionism robs us of so much of our vitality. It tells us we're unworthy. It tells us we aren't allowed to make mistakes, and that when we do we are a failure. It tells us our failures and mistakes make us unlovable. So many lies, yet we believe them!

"Worthy" means: *Having or showing the qualities or abilities that merit recognition in a specified way.*

There are a couple of other words that often cavort with "worthy."

- Deserving

- Enough

What does it mean to deserve something? How do you know you deserve something?

Deserve: Do something, or have or show qualities, worthy of reward or punishment.

We all have privately, perhaps unconsciously built a "worth it" equation for ourselves that explains how we decide whether we are enough of something (but not too much!) to be worthy of deserving something else. Have you ever articulated it?

The blueprint looks like this:

If I am [fill in some qualities or ability], *I will be deserving of (worthy of)* [fill in something you long for].

These sorts of equations often relate to our bodies in some variation on this theme:

If I am thin, I will be deserving of praise.

If I am beautiful, I will be deserving of recognition.

Problem is, we rarely if ever know *what's enough.*

Nothing is ever "good enough" for perfection. There *is* no "skinny enough"; there *is* no "beautiful enough"; there *is* no "kind enough," "strong enough," or "smart enough."

The quest for perfection drives people insane. They lose all perspective. Remember the queen in *Snow White?* She was driven to *murder* to fulfill her quest for perfection!

Mirror, mirror, on the wall,
Who's the fairest of them all?

As it was for her, perfection requires that *you* be the pinnacle of beauty, thinness, virtue, and all the rest of it. And to assess this to be true, perfection scans the world for competition, assesses, compares, and judges. (At least the queen had a magic mirror to do that for her!) But at what cost to you? For the queen, the cost was her sanity and her morality—a steep price! Only *one* person can be the fairest of them all. Perfection requires that you be the *most* thin, the *most* beautiful, the *most* of everything desirable. If you fall short of that expectation—if you're not *enough*—then you are no longer worthy of all the good things in life (especially love), and you *deserve* to be punished.

What's "enough" is a personal decision you make based on your own "worth it" equation.

Take stock right now of the ideals you're invested in. Beauty. Fitness. Thinness. Income earning. Journal on this now, and decide what would be enough of any of them. Title your page "What's Enough?"

1.   How would you know that you had achieved enough?

2.   What would it look like and feel like?

3.   Most importantly, what would you have or experience as a result of attaining enough? What would it make you "deserving of"?

4.   Finally, do you feel like the investment of your time, money, and energy would be *worth it?*

Perfection hurls us into an abyss of perpetual investment, absent clear returns. She takes, but does not give back. It diminishes us. Once we see this, we can make choices that serve us better. Get clear right now and call your energy back for wiser investment.

Imperfection, Failures, and Mistakes

To be human is to be perfectly imperfect.

Perfection is a cruel mistress in so many ways. She doesn't allow for failures and mistakes. She denies us our own essence and our spiritual birthright—to evolve and grow as individuals through mistakes and failures.

You change and grow by trusting yourself enough to make an attempt and risk mistakes or even failure, knowing that you will *survive*. This is how we learn. Trying out new actions and ways of being and making mistakes while you do so is the avenue to growth. When we're busy trying to be perfect, we don't allow ourselves the freedom and the compassion to try and possibly get it wrong or even *flat out fail*.

If you need to loosen perfection's stranglehold on you, know this: The antidote to perfectionism is *play*.

Inscribe an area where you permit yourself to just play and have fun. It doesn't matter if you get it right or even if you are good at the activity. Joyfully mess up! Think right now of three new activities you could take up, where you could allow yourself to be a beginner and get it wrong. Take out your journal and list them right now! Be bold! Go for five! Title your page "Where I'm Free to F*ck Up!"

When we allow ourselves to make mistakes, to get it wrong, and to quickly forgive, we loosen our grip. A loose grip gives us space in which to become. Become what? Something other than what we've been trying desperately to tailor ourselves into. But what might that be? Who is the person who exists outside the bright lines we've engraved with our demands for perfection? She might be a person we don't like, someone we might find

> *The antidote for perfectionism is play.*

unacceptable, shameful, or repugnant. This is a scary thought indeed. Who would you be if you gave up your pursuit of a perfect body?

For the longest time, I believed that I was imperfect and broken beyond repair, a lost cause undeserving of love. Mine would be a loveless existence with a lot of cats. Yep, I was a crazy cat lady—full speed ahead! This vision of myself was, at that time, horrifying. And I pushed her away. She was disgraceful, unacceptable, embarrassing, an awful *mistake* of a human. Do you have a vision of yourself that terrifies you? One of my best friends feared being fat because it embodied all the things about her mother she detested. Being fat isn't a sign of anything definitive. The human living in a fat body has as much right to self-determination as anyone else.

Perfection disallows anything that even seems slightly off the mark. It disowns anything shadowy or triggering. But in murky realms we grow. *No mud; no lotus.*

In retrospect, I can now see what frightened me were actually my own best parts, which I had deemed as unacceptably wild and unfeminine. My hunger for life. My contemplative nature. My mysticism. My empathy for an underdog. My individuality, independence, and intensity. My hermit nature. I could find no archetype of her except as a nun or a witch. In other words: female failures that are social threats. Scary. Now I can see that there is a place for her in my life, one that holds all aspects of me and includes imperfection and love. Accepting this truth has led to a transformation that I believe is truly beautiful, the kind of truthful transformation I wish for you as well.

We're so indoctrinated that mistakes are unacceptable that fear of making one can paralyze us. Journal on these questions. Title your page "Who I'll Be When I Fail."

- What do you fear will happen to you if you mess up?

- What contingencies would you need in place to help you take a risk that might lead to a mistake or even a failure?

- If you failed, how could you forgive yourself?

- What would a failure *allow* for in your life? What pathways would it open?

I believe that your soul yearns for growth—and imperfection, failure, and mistakes are the way! So ponder these questions deeply. When you visualize a woman with all the characteristics you fear the most in yourself, consider for a moment that she might be the most real and authentic version of you. The path to accepting her and making a place for her in your life may be the best reward you ever gain.

Let's check in. After considering the value of mistakes and failures, is your worthiness equation shifting? Are your ideas about "enoughness" changing?

How would you fill this in *now?*

If I am _____ (enough) I will be deserving of (worthy of) _____.

Perhaps go back and journal on this, bearing your new perspective in mind.

Perfection and Love

Each person's "worth it" equation looks a little different, and the aspects of each side are special and unique to them. But I believe most of us yearn to be worthy of the love emanating from another human. The line of reasoning goes like this: perfect body leads to perfect love. *When my body is thinner, stronger, looks better naked, then I will be worthy of love.*

Love is the pinnacle of human experiences. So often when the love we want eludes us, in a search for answers as to *why?* we arrive at simplistic, incorrect conclusions, like we are unlovable because we're fat. We're unlovable because of that gap between the front teeth. We're unlovable because of the thinning hair, the gangly neck, the unusual nose, the acne, or the skin color. Sometimes the criticisms run deeper. We're unlovable because we're *bad.* Our physical flaws are evidence, because we've been taught that good equals beautiful, therefore bad is ugly.

Confronting truth transforms poison into good medicine for your soul.

I have a client who came to the realization she was *relying* on this explanation for everything in her life: *I didn't get the job because they think I'm fat; I didn't get the second date because he thinks I'm fat; they didn't invite me to the party because they think I'm fat; he broke up with me because he thinks I'm fat.* It was only through our work together that she realized *this simply isn't the answer to* everything.

Though vicious, these kinds of conclusions are easier than other, more complex ones that might arise from a more nuanced outlook on life's realities. They're easy because they give us something to control. They're comforting in the face of something that we honestly *don't* comprehend—what love is and how it works. Or even bigger—what *life* is, and how it works. Even if our body-based conclusions are not easy, or even difficult to control, at the very least externalities like freckles and love handles are easy to *blame.*

When we have something to blame, we don't have to do the difficult work, the work that sometimes promises no solid reassurances, conclusions, or answers. Instead, we give ourselves permission to sit and feel victimized by life. It is a victory of the human spirit to recognize that we could choose to feel victimized by the circumstances of our lives and *instead* elect to follow an empowered path. It's an inherently courageous act to engage with the uncertainty of life and, in the face of uncertainty and things that are mostly out of our control, to *still* take fiercely radical responsibility for our thoughts, speech, and behaviors. This is the path of a true spiritual warrior.

Even if we find someone who loves us with our imperfections, we often worry they'll discontinue their love at any moment when they decide to stop overlooking our physical imperfections.

While desire and attraction often turns on an axis of physicality, love shouldn't rely solely on what your body looks like. If someone loves you only because of what you look like, it's not love. If you love yourself because you're pretty, this is not love. Sure, certain faces are prettier to me and I find certain bodies sexier to be intimate with, too, but if that's all that's between me and another person, it's not love.

Love Your Body, Love Your Self

Here's the truth:

Self-love is the only kind of love that we can possibly be guaranteed in this lifetime.

This is why body acceptance is so crucial to our evolution. You cannot love yourself and exclude your body from the circle of love.

No one asked to be here, in this life. You were born against your will. You didn't ask for the body you have. You might quite honestly despise it. But perfection has no space for compassion or forgiveness, and these are exactly the qualities required to accept the body you were given. When we honestly engage with our body that's not as pretty as what we might have ordered up, given the choice; when we treat it with kindness and compassion when it's injured, ill, merely changing, or inevitably growing older, through these merciful acts we learn to "love ourselves." This kind of self-loving impacts all of the other aspects of self housed within. When we make a nourishing home, all parts of our being want to reside there. No longer are you a human looking. No longer are you a human doing. You are now a human being.

Perfection and Purpose

A quest for physical perfection distracts us from the true value in our lives—our dreams, our longings, our heart's desire. These deepest secrets we might share only with the person we trust the most, and maybe not even with that person! When we quest for perfection on the outside, it eases some of the confusion we have about what we are here for. We don't have to look inside at these difficult questions and seek even more complicated answers.

Our life's work is viewed as a "higher calling" or purpose for being alive. The yogis believe that our presence on earth is not random, but purposeful. We are all warriors on the battlefields of our own lives, engaged in the path of the hero, on a hero's journey. It's intriguing to view life this way.

We could decide we're just here to pay our bills and watch TV. The choice is ours. It's almost easier to believe that we're here for no reason. It absolves us of any responsibility. From that vantage point, we have time to waste. We can destroy our planet, the living beings on it, and our relationships—nothing matters. But if you decide that life is worth something—*you* are worth something—well then you have no time to lose setting about figuring out why you are here. And in light of that, we may find that our physical appearance becomes far less important, and our thoughts and actions increase in worth. And in this way, we take radical responsibility for ourselves—who we are, what we are, what we believe in and stand for.

Thích Nhất Hạnh teaches that our only true belongings are our actions.[18] We're led to believe that we own our bank account, our possessions, and even our body. But those things could easily disappear. Even if we attained the physical perfection that we are seeking, it could dissolve slowly, via aging, or swiftly, in a car accident. In the end you will be remembered for how you made people feel and what you did to improve their lives.

When I arrived in New York, for a moment I thought that I really wanted to be a model. I was still consumed by the body/beauty value equation. Nothing else was right in my life—but at least I could be thin! But, as I thought about it, the high hourly wage I might have commanded didn't seem to be "worth it." I didn't want to "waste my time" being photographed when I could instead spend it creating ideas, teaching, educating, and affecting other people in the pursuit of values that were and are truer to my being. I wanted to be remembered for the bravery of my actions and the impact I had in improving other people's lives.

In the end, you will be remembered for how you made people feel and what you did to improve their lives.

Our true longings, our heart's desire, our life's work are so tender, so vulnerable, so precious, and so often seemingly remote and out of reach, like a dream, that we tend to armor them over with more concrete and easily understandable pursuits, like a quest for physical perfection. In a world where everything seems so uncontrollable, at the very least we can take charge of the plan to get in shape! Or to home decorate! Or to get a new car! We seek to control what little we can.

But is it what your heart truly yearns for?

As I learned about the idea of *life's work* or *higher calling* and started to consider what my life might be used for, I concluded that, fundamentally, humans are here to alleviate the suffering of other humans and all other living beings. We are here to learn to love better.

It is the human condition to suffer. As brothers and sisters to our fellow humans, we can either heap it on or help dissipate it. When we take the poison of a person's suffering and alter it for the better, that is alchemy of the highest order. That is good medicine.

We all come into the world naked and free of all money and possessions. We will leave the world the same way. What happens in your heart, what actions you take while you are here—these are the sum value of your life. These are your true worth and value.

Finding your way is a path littered with missteps and mistakes. It will be "imperfect." And that is exactly what will make it truly beautiful.

WHAT DOES YOUR SOUL YEARN FOR?

According to the yogis, it's no accident we're here, alive, on earth. Life is a journey of discovery, a transformation, and the soul's evolution. As Joseph Campbell calls it, "the hero's journey." It's heroic because it requires bravery.

Growth doesn't come without confrontation; that's the nature of things. If evolving were easy, everyone would be doing it! Finding out what you're here to do with your one precious life is a *practice*.

To find out what we really want—not what the animal part of us wants, which is sleep, food, and sex, but what the *soul* or *spirit* part of us wants—we must connect to our hearts.

This is why the "heart log" assignment that I gave you in the core practice of Lesson 2 is very important. It is the tool that you need for this next assignment. If you don't recall it or haven't been doing it, go back and review!

In yoga, there's a practice to help find out why we're here, to sustain our efforts, and to help us assess the results. I mentioned it in Lesson 1; the practice is called sankalpah. Sankalpah means, roughly, "heart's desire" or "heartfelt resolve." Our resolve is crucial because it signifies our deep commitment to stick with our life choices.

A sankalpah helps us to connect our heart's desire to the day-to-day elements of our lives, so we can create bigger outcomes we can feel proud of. When you adopt daily practices and do *everything* with intention, it will profoundly affect and change the course of your life.

There are three kinds of sankalpah: intent for the day, intent for the phase of life, and intent for your dharma or life's work.

Here's a sankalpah I've been working with recently:

"I am love; I feel love; I receive love."

I crafted this in response to my belief that the great work of my life, my *dharma,* is about repairing love, in myself, in my family, and in the people around me. These statements express longings of incredible proportions. My life commitment is huge. Yours might be too!

I have a group of students, in New York City and around the world, who are committed to sankalpah as a practice of engaging with their life and experience. Here are some of theirs they offered to share with you.

"I am a gentle, caring soul."

"I share myself with grace, equanimity, and fearlessness."

"I have the strength to love."

"The strength to open my heart to love is within me."

"I make healthy choices."

"I speak with patience and compassion to my loved ones."

A sankalpah could also relate to the phase of life that you are in, working to support you in a specific time period. Here are a few that represent this idea:

"I am financially solvent and I am enough."

"I am in a loving sustainable relationship with a reliable and supportive partner."

And here are some from my yoga-teacher colleagues here in New York City that represent sankalpah to support daily action:

"I eat healthier."

"I am compassionate."

"I inspire through my actions."

"I seek solutions."

"I am calm in the midst of chaos."

"I do my laundry with joy."

"I remain grounded in the present moment."

"I meditate five minutes a day."

"I cultivate healthier bonds with others."

"I find joy in my work."

"I nurture myself; I nurture others."

"I find the silver lining in each cloud."

"I am present when with others."

"I am strong/loveable/light/patient/tolerant/forgiving/spontaneous/relaxed..."

Here are some that relate specifically to the body:

"I am at home in my body."

"My body is wise beyond knowing."

"Movement is my medicine."

"I trust my body to know what's best for me."

"My body is a safe harbor for my spirit."

"I free myself from critical thoughts toward my body and worth."[19]

"I am on a path to knowing and trusting my body's wisdom."

To review, a sankalpah can help you with a daily intention, a phase of life intention, or a dharma intention. No matter its purpose, the most basic and essential element of the sankalpah is that it's written in present tense. The core understanding of reality is that *everything you need is already here now and you already are everything that you require to have the kind of life you want.* This is based on an understanding of time—the only thing that exists is *now* and contained in *now* is *all* of time. The past. The present. The future. It all exists only and ever *now.* Our sense that time is linear is a misperception. It's a way that we humans make sense of and organize our experiences that is commensurate with our human (as opposed to "divine") capacity to perceive. Our limited minds cannot contain all of eternity, so we manage by deluding ourselves into thinking time is linear. This makes it manageable.

With the present-tense formation (only, ever, *now),* statements like "I want to be more compassionate" become "Compassion is my true nature" or "I am compassion itself."

Or "I will not eat fried food" becomes "With compassion for my body and for other beings, I eat a clean diet."

These statements of heartfelt desire are the small building blocks that will take us toward the answer to the larger, and sometimes overwhelming, question of "What am I here for?" and keep us on track to becoming the best rendition of ourselves. Just as it's unwise to go out and run a marathon without first having put in a few miles, it's not a great idea to tackle that *big* question without first addressing smaller ones. If we don't do the smaller pieces first, chances are we'll feel overwhelmed and just give up.

Do this now: Look at your heart log. Notice what sorts of themes emerge with the most frequency.

They will probably fall into one of two categories:

- A longing that reflects your true nature

- An intention or goal that reflects your true nature

Pull these out, and see if you can draft a sankalpah. You'll have opportunities to revise, redirect, even throw it out and start all over again! You are not shackled to this—it doesn't need to be perfect.

The practice of sankalpah is merely a process of discovering and then purposefully directing your thoughts about yourself. It's all an experiment. What you think is important, so take the time to decide what you *want* to think.

HOW TO USE YOUR SANKALPAH INTENTION

You already know the answer to this! Do a movement practice with it in mind—run, swim, do yoga! It's important what you think while you move. You can meditate—sitting, walking, breathing—while focusing on it. Whenever I find an empty space in my day, I think about mine. Sometimes I even think about it when I'm asleep! Part of its power is in its potential to fill up the space we ordinarily fill with garbage thoughts, or self-deprecating thoughts, or comparative thoughts, or judgmental thoughts. The power of using your body in concert with your sankalpah is that it creates a resonance between your thoughts and your body and allows you to access the wisdom of your body *about* your life's purpose. Actually engaging with and using your body is the key to unlocking its messages for you!

The heartfelt desire and the resolve of sankalpah spill into a greater calling—dharma or *life's work*. The basic idea is that when you work intentionally on your resolve a little bit every day, those tiny strands join

What you do today matters most!

together to make yarn that weaves into a bigger tapestry yet—the great work of your life.

Remember, your sankalpah doesn't have to be perfect! You get to play, experiment, make mistakes, revise, learn, and grow. Enjoy yourself! Whatever you do, be playful, make mistakes, forgive yourself fast, and begin again. This is the way we disarm perfectionism and reclaim our right to learn, grow, and evolve.

Your body is an essential part of your mystical toolkit for the evolution of your soul. When we waste precious time in the perfection project, we poison ourselves and lose energy, which we could otherwise pull back into the present moment and spend on a breakthrough. Without access to the vital information from your body, you're fragmented and functioning at a disadvantage. When you skillfully use your body and the wisdom it possesses, what was once a world of black and white will become full color. Your senses come alive, and the garden of your life springs into bloom. I so want this vivid living to be available to you, dear reader! Freeing yourself from the perfection project is a huge part of living authentically and brilliantly.

Now, I have some good news for you: you've made it through much of the most difficult material. Hurray! The lessons that follow are, in many ways, far easier than those you've just learned. While the garden pathway of your life will always present weeds and boulders, these obstacles will be *so much easier* to contend with now that you've got the crucial mind-set shifts from lessons 1 through 3. Congratulations! Let's forge ahead, armed with your new, helpful thoughts. Machetes at the ready...

The body is the shore on the ocean of being.

—Sufi (anonymous)

LESSON 4

Tame the Spin Doctor (The Power of Choice)

I've mentioned that a few years ago I found I had gained about twenty pounds. Indoctrinated as I was then in the inherent social value of being thin, this was bad.

Let's look at this situation from some other people's perspective.

For the clothes designers, manufacturers, and distributors, the fact that I'd gained enough weight that my clothes and bras no longer fit was a good thing, because it meant that I would have to buy new items to fit this different body.

For the owners of places of fitness—gyms or yoga studios—this weight gain was a good thing, because it meant that I was more likely to enroll in a membership and exercise, freshly invested in a weight-loss project.

For the proprietors of bookstores, or those who run online media outlets, the weight gain was a good thing, because it meant that I was more likely to come in and purchase some materials about weight loss or health, or even purchase some equipment to attain those things.

For a romantic interest, my weight gain could be a good thing, if he preferred a person with a meatier body and bigger breasts. Or it could be a bad thing if he didn't like living with a person who was a bit depressed.

For the medical industry, my weight gain could be viewed as a good thing if eventually it led me to need their care.

So, for many people, my weight gain would actually be a good event. They stood to make some money.

In fact, for many *more* people than me, it would be a good thing. I was perhaps the only person who might view it as a bad thing. So which was it? Good? Bad?

Neither. *It's empty of significance.*

Also, consider this: my decision that it's bad could be misplaced. What if I simply changed my mind?

Because what if, through this "bad" weight gain, I suddenly became a plus-size model, and gained a contract with an agency? Cha-ching!

What if, through this "bad" weight gain, I attracted the attention of a man who really prefers a woman with meat on her bones, and we fell in love and realized that—wow!—we were a terrific match?

What if, through this weight gain, I came to inspire many students who feel out of place in yoga classes, because they think that yoga is just for already skinny people?

What if this became a real strength for my teaching? What if it became the cornerstone of my yoga teaching and the most important part of my business model?

What if I decided that I prefer wearing a 32-F bra size? What if I found that having big breasts is an attribute that I could wield to my advantage?

What if I decided that being heavier is actually *just fine* with me? What if? What if? *What if?*

Now, is this weight gain a good thing, or a bad thing?

Who knows? And not knowing what the outcome may be—when a purportedly bad circumstance arises —is exactly the hidden potential in *all* circumstances. But so often, we decide in advance we already know if something is good or bad, and this creates a state of mind that is either unrealistically gloomy or optimistic.

Have you ever had an experience in which you thought something horrible happened, and when you looked back you could see that actually is had a blessing inside?

It is quite possible that things could turn out far better than we had imagined.

Here's one thing we *can* know for sure, about the body, thinness, and its relationship to commerce. In the now iconic words of Naomi Wolf:

> A culture fixated on female thinness is not an obsession about female beauty, but an obsession about female obedience. Dieting is the most potent political sedative in women's history; a quietly mad population is a tractable one.[20]

When people are starving, they cannot think clearly. When people cannot think clearly, they will often believe what they are told, and behave as they are asked to: *this is good; that is bad; do this, not that.* Some people will think that you are smart, beautiful, and important. Others will disagree. Ultimately, it's not important what they think. What's important is what *you* think. (Did I mention that it's hard to think when you're chronically hungry?) What you think about yourself is entirely your choice. If you think it's good, it's good. If you think it's bad, it's bad. Fundamental responsibility for ourselves belongs to us, and us alone. You get to be the kind of woman you want to be. How exciting! Challenge the role models you have been spoon-fed. Tell yourself your own story about who you are and who you are destined to be. Spin the events of your life into empowering narratives. But first, ya gotta stop starving yourself!

GOOD AND BAD DON'T EXIST

All events are empty of significance. This can be very hard to grasp. But what about the Holocaust? What about starvation in Africa? Surely these events are *bad* or even *evil!* Essentially, the question here is "Why do bad things happen?" Try telling the person in the concentration camp that "events are empty of significance," and surely that argument will not augur well.

A yogic explanation suggests that every being is a manifestation of the divine, a way for it to be embodied and therefore to experience *all* that life has to offer. The divine doesn't discriminate, doesn't select only good experiences. It wants to have them all. It wants to experience them *all*. The rapturous. The horrifying. The joyous. The miserable. Ecstasy. Bliss. Wrath. Rage. *Everything.* To the universe, all experiences are equally worth having. Good and bad are human inventions.

Families and Spin

We're all subjected to broad social structures of what is designated good and bad, and to more granular renditions within our families of origin. When we were children, choice and interpretation were not ours to command. We wore the clothes our parents bought us, ate the foods that they introduced us to, listened to the words that they spoke. We absorbed their ideas of what is good and what is bad. Because it was all that we knew, we integrated it as real, normal, and true. Our parents were gods.

When we're young, we usually subscribe to our parents' ideals, along with other agreements, like those we make with schools, government, religions. Growing up, we start to get a bigger picture. We see what other people wear and eat and how they talk. We have something to compare with our formative experiences. At this juncture we're presented with choice. Maturing, it's our responsibility to examine these beliefs and either confirm them or deny them.

You now have an abundance of information about *why* we've been taught to think about our bodies the way that we have, and we'll continue to explore this further. Becoming an adult, you have options; you can *choose* what to believe. But, now you face a real challenge, because the most difficult thing in the world is to change your own mind. To do so, you must persist in change, and growth, *especially* when confronted with information that challenges the way that you've become accustomed to seeing the world. Your willingness to entertain ideas that don't fit nicely with what you already believe takes courage. It requires a warrior's heart. Good for you for choosing! It is the path of the evolving soul.

The most difficult thing in the world is to change your own mind.

The Spin Doctor: That's You!

Just as nothing can be absolutely perfect, nothing can be good or bad. For good and bad to be universal, everyone must agree—and people simply don't. We all are little spin doctors. Countless times daily we decide whether things are good or bad. Impartiality or an absence of bias simply does not exist. As your mind stretches out into the world, it likes to formulate judgments. That's how the mind knows it's real. It has a thought about something. *I think, therefore I am.* Its own body is the first thing of material significance the mind encounters in the world. Therefore, to understand its own positioning in the world, the mind likes to create opinions, judgments, and relativities— *I'm prettier than that person. This is a good thing.* It's comforting to know where we stand, but certainty can also shut out possibility.

All events are essentially empty of meaning, and therefore full of potential. This is the hidden potential in all things. Is that an obstacle before you? Or is it actually an opportunity? It's a matter of perspective and the mind's flexibility.

Teacher Geshe Michael Roach says that despite the fact that all events are blank, or neutral, or "empty," we don't experience them as such. We *experience* them as having some significance, and we attribute that significance to something outside of ourselves. Geshe Roach writes:

> And yet, we do experience some things as good things, and we do experience other things as bad things. If it's not coming from the things themselves, then where is it coming from? If we could solve this puzzle, then perhaps we could *make things happen the way we wanted them to.*
>
> It's pretty obvious with just a few moments of reflection that the way we see things *is coming from ourselves.*[21]

This is a high level of radical responsibility for our own experience, to admit it emanates from us! It's so much easier to *blame*— people, society, the world, the weather, our parents—the list can be so long! When you think though your life, surely there are places where you could start to shift your spin and perspective. You can take responsibility for your perceptions in so many areas: health, your body, family, work, friendships, partnerships, and small interactions with people all throughout the day. Does one of these call you to an opportunity for a shift in perspective? We're working on how we feel about the body, but a different area may resonate more. Go with that first instinct!

Sometimes it feels good to blame other people for our experiences. Sometimes it's all we know how to do, because we've not been taught to see things any other way. You can start taming your spin doctor with a wonderful practice from Thích Nhất Hạnh. When you're sure that someone is out to get you, or something totally sucks, stop these perceptions by asking, "Am I sure?"[22] Write *Are you sure?* on a sticky note. Put it somewhere you will see it often as a reminder to check your spin.

I sometimes use this technique along with one more step. As a follow-up to "Are you sure?" I'll ask my client or myself "How do you know?" Often we'll discover that the answer is built on conjecture about another's feelings, or speculation about their motive, or some confining notion of "how the world works." You could never hope to fully and completely understand how others think or feel, and "the way the world works" is always open to interpretation. We know very little about how others feel, and it's completely out of our control. It's important what *you* think or feel. You can adjust your thoughts and feelings to your advantage. In the words of Nelson Mandela—a person who *surely* could have spun his situation badly—"It always seems impossible until it's done." This is the power of choice, to choose what we think and believe. This power is available to you! You need only to decide.

HELPING YOUR SPIN DOCTOR WHEN THE BODY INEVITABLY DISAPPOINTS

It might happen you're caught so deeply in wrong perceptions that it's difficult to choose a different way of looking at the situation.

Sometimes, it takes others introducing new ideas to really have them take root.

When it comes to the body we tend to be rigid.

Weigh more? *Bad.*

Weigh less? *Good.*

Mom bod? *Bad.*

Pre-baby body? *Good.*

Looking older, wrinkles, grey hair? *Bad.*

Looking younger? *Good.*

Illness, injury, or other major unwanted changes? *Bad. Definitely bad.*

Things can't possibly be so black and white. You have other options! You just might need them pointed out. Let's look at some fresh ways to view these topics.

Aging

A few years ago grey hairs began collecting along my part line. I mentioned this to one of my best girls, Ann, and in response she surprised me by crooning "preeettyyyy!" As she is someone I trust and respect, I was interested in her opinion. She helped me shift perspective about the physical beauty of aging, and thus the value of an older woman.

In most societies there is a natural place for older men and women. It is the place of "wisdom keeper." Our wise elders have their own life experience and also hold institutional knowledge of society and traditions. Their time for active production is past; now their contribution is to hold the wisdom and share it when it is needed, like a human library.

Our own society no longer values the wisdom of our elders—especially elder women. They view them as a burden. We're taught to value youth in multiple layers of human interactions—first-hand, through our mothers, and through advertising and marketing and media. It broke my heart when I saw my mother mourning the loss of her youth, but it also educated me.

Feminist Silvia Federici documents the relationship between one of the largest, least talked about genocides in the history of humanity—the witch hunts—and its relationship to the transition between feudalism and capitalism. In their role as wisdom keepers, older women and childless women remembered how things were before the peasantry's common lands were taken away from them and privatized. These women protested and reminded people how things used to be. An efficient way to cleanse the memory of the populace is to criminalize and exterminate those who *remember*. This is one of the many reasons that witches became portrayed as old, or childless, or ugly. It was *old* people who recalled the past, and that it was then better for people. Disney has memorialized these tropes visually, indoctrinating children with stories and images of witches as outcast, evil, often childless, usually ugly, old women.

Our mothers are our first real connection with having a female body and also to an aging female body. Our mothers often inadvertently teach us to hate ourselves because *they* were taught to hate themselves.

Examples abound of how our mothers miseducated us. One of my colleagues recounts being cat-called while walking home, and how it made her feel unsafe. She told her mother, anticipating comfort. Instead she was told "That's the price of being a woman." One of my client's foundational teachings from her mother was that if she was fat, people wouldn't like her, so she put her on a diet as an eight-year-old. My own mother taught me to fear my body and its sexuality, and to cover up my cleavage.

What different lives all of us would have if we were instead taught to respect our bodies, protect our sexuality, and wield both well. As we work together, my clients come to see that in most cases our mothers did what they thought was right and what they thought would keep us safe. You might not be able to perceive that yet, but I believe that you too will see this, especially as you move into a time of life as a mentor, leader, or elder. You'll see that you are doing the best you can with the tools on hand. You might notice those tools are insufficient for the task before you, but the kinds of resources you truly need are so much more available today than they were for our mothers. In a time when it's commonly understood that problematic childhood beliefs are often formed at our parents' hands, these realizations have helped me forgive my own mother. She did the best she knew how. We are so very lucky to be alive right now! I wish wholeheartedly that my mother had at her disposal the information and tools presently so readily available. I bet it could have helped her, as a woman, and also eased her parenting challenges.

Clients often come to my coaching because they realize they're inadvertently modeling their own legacy of self-hatred to their children, just as their mothers did for them. One powerful commitment you can make today as you model being the wisest version of yourself is to never, ever speak disparagingly about your body or any other woman's body. Pledge to speak kindly of yourself, at all costs.

Let's begin to celebrate aging, and being old. To counteract damaging narratives, let's create new ones. I've started to envision myself with a crown of platinum hair. I've realized this is just one piece of having a beautiful vision of myself as a mature woman. To have that, I am the one who needs to hold this image in my mind and heart. When every one of us holds that vision for ourselves, we also help other women who are having difficulty escaping that "old is bad and young is good" spin.

Pledge to speak kindly of yourself, at all costs.

In fact, thinking well about aging isn't just a nice idea: it's proven to have positive outcomes. A Yale University Study found that in a group of 4,765 people with an average age of seventy-two, those who carried a gene variant linked to dementia—but also had positive attitudes about aging—were 50 percent less likely to develop the disorder than people who carried the gene but faced aging with more pessimism or fear.[23] Our bodies are less likely to disappoint when we think well about them.

Is greying hair a good thing or a bad thing? It's neither. As a sign of aging, it has only the value you assign and the story you choose to tell yourself about it. Begin to notice older women you especially admire.

Take out your journal now, and write from these prompts and questions. Title your page "Aging Admiration."

- What is it that inspires you about these older women? Who is an "older woman" role model for you?

- What are some great things about getting older? You can ask this of the women around you. Start to create a picture today of the woman you want to be as you age.

- When you think of your older, wiser self, what does she look like, move like, speak like? What does she wear, who does she spend time with, what does she do? What kinds of emotions does she experience? If you don't know, begin to craft that for yourself today!

Consider this visioning a kind and generous gesture to the future you, positioning her to be the best version of herself that she can. Choose ways of thinking that help you to feel authentically good about yourself. This will restore your power *and* that of the people around you. What a wonderful, kind gift to yourself and everyone you interact with!

Illness

Along with aging, illness is another likely, probably disappointing inevitability. At age forty-two my friend and colleague Kelley Rush was diagnosed with breast cancer, had a double mastectomy, and elected not to have her breasts reconstructed.

Cancer of any form is, for many, a worst-case scenario. For most women, losing their breasts is another, compounded nightmare. Kelley's decision not to have them rebuilt was in greatest service to her health, but this certainly did not come without a tremendous sense of loss for her and her immensely supportive husband. Luckily, Kelley is now in remission.

When I asked if she would describe her illness as good or bad, she laughed and said, "Depends on the day and what I'm thinking about!"

Kelley described her experience in terms of down days and up days, but in broad brushstrokes, she said that overall the experience has been *good*. She gave two top reasons for her assessment:

- Cancer prompted her to reprioritize her life each day, and to ask herself *Do I have my priorities straight or at least in line with my vision?*

- Facing death drove her to not waste a single day of her precious life and to live in alignment with the best of her intentions in the best and positive way.

We all seem to think that we have plenty of time; we think that we have more time than we do. Our bodies will die, and our lives are a treasure—we should make the most of them, every day!

Kelley noticed that having urgency about living can create its own set of problems on down days. On days that she feels tired and wants to give her body a rest, another voice speaks up: "Don't waste even one more day; get up!" Some of this was also fueled by the loss of two friends to cancer, and survivor's guilt. She mused out loud, "How come I got to live, while they died?"

During her illness, Kelley used her skillful body relationship that she had cultivated through decades of yoga practice. She continued to practice yoga as she was able. Sometimes stretching her fingers *was* her yoga practice. She found support and help adjusting to the new reality of "being flat" through online communities. She made the decision to let her breasts go with the complete support of her husband, who also, of course, mourned their departure. Men bond with our breasts! It's impossible to say that her relationship with her body *ensured* her survival, but I believe that her skillfulness in working with it, forgiving it, feeling compassion for it went far in helping her to ease her own pain, sadness, fear, and disappointment throughout the experience. In the end, her deep internal work, viewing her body as a sacred vessel for her spirit, created the possibility for her to, in her own words, sur-*thrive!*

In addition to these supportive steps, Kelley also volunteers once a year in Eleuthera, in the Bahamas, teaching yoga to women who have had mastectomies. This is one of the greatest self-help techniques when our spin doctor gets out of control and tells us everything is *baaaaaad*—to be helpful to others. It gets us out of our heads and helps us to see the world from a different perspective.

When you're having a down day—it doesn't need to be about an illness, necessarily, it could just be about life—look for ways to get out of your own head. Call a friend, or do something helpful for another person, or just show a kindness to anyone around you. These small acts help us shift our perceptions and also our feelings.

One reason I believe that a good body relationship is imperative is because it will better prepare us for the inevitability of an illness. When we confront an illness—especially one that threatens our survival—we come face to face with who we really are and the value of our own lives. Are we good to our bodies, and are we living our best lives? These become priority questions. Start to take stock of this in small ways and get out ahead of these questions. Don't wait for a tragedy! Are you good to your body? When you have a cold, perhaps you just push through and go to work. Maybe it's time to address *why* you do that, and put in place structures allowing your body to heal when it is sick. Maybe you don't sleep enough, eat often enough or healthy enough foods; maybe you drink too much coffee or alcohol and not enough water. Your health depends most of what you do every day. Now is the best time to make a change!

Your health depends most on what you do every day.

These are the first steps toward learning to take care of your body so that when you're more seriously compromised you have a good foundation to build on to help yourself. You don't need to wait for an illness. You can also teach yourself a new way when you're working with an injury.

Injury

We're accustomed to thinking that injury is a bad thing, for so many understandable reasons. It hurts! It slows us down! It's inconvenient. We have to change our plans, in the moment, perhaps in the future, and maybe forever!

Most people have some kind of active or latent injury. Take stock of your own body right now. How many old injuries do you have? Got any active ones talking to you? When we're injured (or ill!), that is the moment we need our good relationship with our bodies the most. If you're used to relating to your body through movement, and then hurt yourself and can no longer do that movement, it can feel as if you've been exiled from your most intimate relationship. This is the very time that your body needs you to be *in* it, seeking ways to stay connected, breathing, feeling, supporting it. Do not abandon your body when it gets hurt! When you get hurt—which inevitably will happen—think about how you can continue your movement practices and stay connected to your body and therefore to yourself.

Teaching yoga, I'm often surprised that my students disappear when they get hurt. We need our yoga more than ever when we're hurt! These students have not been taught how to adapt their practice for every situation. Yoga is one of the most malleable body practices; when taught by the right teacher it's suitable for people of any age or ability. When we teach yoga only to the young, fit, able, healthy, and uninjured, we are missing most of the population.

My private yoga practice in New York City is all about supporting these people and helping them feel better in and about their bodies. When the body feels like a constant disappointment—not for any cosmetic reason, but because of how it's hindering your lifestyle and enjoyment of life—that's when you most urgently need support in getting back in touch with it.

At a holiday party this year, a guest said to me, "I can't do yoga right now—I have a

When we teach yoga only to the young, fit, able, healthy, and uninured, we are missing most of the population.

concussion." And *that* was my entry into a discussion about the many ways to adapt the practice for her injury to help her stay in contact with her body throughout the healing process, and also to assist in the experience. She is now my client.

Not *all* my classroom students disappear when they get hurt. One of my students, Lisa, a medical doctor, showed up one day with a cast on her arm. She had broken her wrist. Though I was bummed out for her, I was absolutely *thrilled* that she knew she could come to my class in a cast, trusting that I have the skills to take care of her and help her find ways to make the practice work.

Lisa assessed the injury as a good thing. She reported that it gave her fresh perspective and appreciation for her overall health. For many people, an injury is a forced slowdown, a moment to evaluate how you've been doing things. It's almost like life intervenes and makes you take a pause. For Lisa, the injury helped her be more patient with herself.

Lisa said, "The injury really got me in touch with my body in such a strong way. I became much less concerned about how others perceived my body and more about my internal body awareness. It truly helped with my body image as I am so much more grateful for having a body that serves me in so many capacities. The injury was a challenge, a grace, and a blessing."

The next time you get hurt, how can you think about your injury? Can you view it as an opportunity for growth? Are there injuries that you experience repeatedly? I was talking with a client of mine about the instances when she sprains her ankles. It's almost *always* right after the thought *I need to slow down!* I also hurt my feet often. I know that these instances are moments when I'm growing inside at a pace that is just a bit faster than other parts of me would like. The injury is a way to sabotage that growth. Injury is literal and also mystical.

Injury is literal and also mystical.

At every juncture—with injury, illness, aging—we can choose how to think about our bodies and our experience within them. We can decide if it's good or bad.

We can decide if it's mundane or it's mystical. We can decide if it's a little of all of the above.

And you can also decide it all sucks, because that's a real part of the truth too. Things are rarely all good or all bad, all basic or all complex, all black or all white. We live in a world of so many shades of grey.

OTHER PEOPLE ARE SPIN DOCTORS TOO

Sometimes the people around us help us create new, healthy perceptions. Other times they entrench old perceptions that perpetuate suffering. It can be difficult *not* to get caught up in the opinions of others. And it can be hard when you're forming new ideas about your body and your self. I want you to be resilient to other people's spin. No matter whether others' opinions contain praise or judgment, grow to be so solid in yourself that you hold steady through anything. Know thyself.

Nevertheless, it can be hard not to be affected by others' thoughts and emotions.

Because I'm a yoga instructor, my body is constantly on display. When I lose weight, people say, "Wow! You're looking quite lean!" They smile and clearly approve. It's difficult not to get caught up in this. Even if I disagree with the premise, having the approval of others feels so good! But the flip side is, I'll also get entangled in the silence and disapproval around any weight gain. I refuse this agreement.

Even if other people cannot see your value, that doesn't erase its existence.

A colleague noted that I was looking lean in the face. I said, "I am lean! But next week, I might be plump, so there's no use in getting too caught up in it!" He laughed, understanding my position.

Check yourself when you feel the momentary high from others' approval. When you accept that hit, you give away your power. Your power resides in the knowledge that you're valuable with or without anyone else's approval. You are valuable for simply being. You need not deflect others' approval or use the moment to seek additional compliments. All you need to do is say "Thank you!" and move along.

Growing up, and waking up, means you get to make up your own mind! Think your own thoughts. Be your own person! Start with the way that you think about your body, its worth, and therefore *your* intrinsic value. The way you think about your body—its weight gain, loss, aging, wrinkling, relative health or sickness—is entirely a matter of your perception, and beginning to reason differently will change the way you measure the value of your life. One thing we know for sure—the body will grow sick and die. You can create your own relationship with this inevitability. Take care of the body, and cultivate who you *are*. Your *being*. Choose what to believe. No one else can select for you. There's simply no reason not to choose empowering thoughts! Surround yourself with people who are on the same kind of quest. When you go with friends and allies, you will go far.

Spin Interventions

When people want to spin things—whether about you or about others—in a direction you think isn't helpful or healthy, it's wise to be armed with clever diversionary tactics.

There are two big categories of spin: creating it and receiving it.

Creating Spin: Talking About Others

Talking about others can be a healthy way to process the events of our lives. Other people's actions affect us, impact us, and create feelings.

Sometimes talking about others amounts to nothing more than gossip. How can you tell which it is?

Here are some ways to identify gossip.

- Does it reinforce—or punish the lack of—morality and accountability?

- Does it reveal passive aggression, isolating and harming others?

- Does it serve as a process of social grooming?

- Does it build and maintain a sense of community with shared interests, information, and values?

- Does it begin a courtship that helps one find their desired mate, by counseling others?

- Does it provide a peer-to-peer mechanism for disseminating information?

Gossip often just *feels* yucky. To know if it's a helpful or harmful discussion of another person check in with how it feels. If it feels gross, in any way, make an effort to stop. If it feels clean, and free of any energetic charge, proceed with caution. Here are some basic tips for handling gossip.

- Pull your energy back into the present moment, with the people you're actually with.

- Insist on talking about only the people present in the room: *their lives, their concerns.*

- If you are talking about another person, make sure it is used to help you have insights into your own life and experiences.

- Make it part of your ethics to only speak well of people when they are not around, particularly if they have done nothing to harm you personally.

- Combat gossip by countering with kind, generous, compassionate statements. Insist that you do not know the entire story as to why a person speaks or behaves the way they do. Never rob another person of their autonomy. Make space for them to speak for themselves.

Here's a quote to live by: *Gossip ends at a wise person's ear.*

Handling Spin About You

Some people just can't stop themselves. They *have* to comment on your body!

I think it's useful to have rehearsed, gracious, de-escalating responses to incendiary remarks, like the following:

- "It looks like you've gained weight!" *Haha! Maybe! My body does what it does. By the way: You look* wonderful! *I love you so much, and I'm so happy to see you. What is something really terrific that has happened to you recently?*

- "You look so great! Have you lost weight?" *I'm not sure! I don't weigh myself. I really try to not get caught up in that: it makes me crazy and ends up taking up so much of my mental space, space that I want to spend thinking about truly important things. Speaking of really important things, how is your [fill in the blank—choose something you know is really important to that person in their life] going?*

My mock responses aim to help you point out how rarely what we have, or don't have, in the looks department has anything to do with *us personally.* You were born into a body you did not select. The body truly has a mysterious and magical life of its own—what it does, and why, we can hardly fathom. We are empowered to affect areas like our personality, degree of kindness, and ability to learn, change, and grow. When you respond skillfully to body comments, you have the opportunity to educate the people around you and to elevate the human condition overall, to emphasize valuing what's inside over what's outside, and to abide in a place where things aren't clearly good or bad. You can prethink these sorts of scenarios and plan gracious escapes for yourself and for the other person. These conversations often have a contracting sensation, so quest for an expansive feeling. You might feel trapped. Trust your heart to tell you when you've landed on a solution that feels honest, generous, and kind for all people involved.

Choosing for Things to Be Bad

Have you ever been around a person for whom everything is always bad? What does it feel like? How does it impact them? How does it impact you? If you're presented the option to suffer or not—which you almost always are—how do you choose?

You may have heard this saying: "Pain is certain; suffering is optional."

The medical intuitive, mystic, and author Caroline Myss coined a term for the frame of mind for people who are disproportionately committed to their suffering: "woundology." This pathology arises when we overidentify with the pain of the circumstances and create an identity around it. Our traumas, our misfortunes, our illnesses, our body's virtues or failings: our circumstances become *who we are.* These attachments can cause suffering.

If you really dig deep and realize that you are in fact unwilling to give up your bad spin, or your suffering, be extremely kind with yourself. There are probably complicated reasons for your commitment to your suffering. Begin to wonder, *Well, what is that reason? Why would I actually* want *to go on suffering like this?*

I've identified four main reasons:

1. The first is easy—if we choose to suffer, everything is someone else's fault and we have a wonderful escape from taking responsibility for our perceptions. We're passive victims of the world's injustices. It's someone else's fault!

2. Having something to suffer over makes us feel special. When we suffer, it creates a reason for other people to interact with us, to give us their time, compassion, attention, sympathy.

3. The third reason is much more complex, ironically, in a very simple way. Change is scary and uncomfortable, and we *never* know exactly what will come from it. Often when presented with the option to continue suffering an ill that we are familiar with, versus moving toward a different experience that we

have no familiarity with, we will probably choose to stay with what we know.

4. Finally, if we choose to change, it means that *we have to take ultimate, radical responsibility for our own experiences*. And *that*, my friend, is a lot of hard, but rewarding, work.

Chances are you will choose change only when you've suffered sufficiently to reach your breaking point. This moment is filled with tremendous power, because at that moment you have tons of energy, and practically anything is possible. Are you ready to choose change? I'll anticipate your answer is yes. Putting a new spin on things is the first step. What follows is a step-by-step process to plant the seeds for change.

TRANSFORM YOUR SPIN DOCTOR INTO A CHANGE AGENT

Here's a simple way to experience change. Put down any instrument you're writing with. Now pick it up with your other hand and write your name.

That's change. Awkward. Uncomfortable. Uncertain. Out of control!

Your ability to change is built on the truths of your life. Some of you have moved from one continent to another. Some of you have had children and built families. Others have changed careers and jobs. You've survived breakups, deaths in the family, and heartaches. This is evidence that you are more than capable of making and enduring change. If you ever doubt it, remind yourself of these core truths. And, now, make a choice to change the spin that you put on the events of your life, and specifically around your body and your relationship with it.

Ana Forrest has an effective Formula for Change[24] that you can call upon when you find yourself about to create a spin.

1. Catch that you are doing the behavior.

2. Take ten deep breaths and reset.

3. Reward yourself lavishly for catching the behavior.

4. Take one step toward healing.

These steps seem simple, but they *will* take practice!

Step One: Catch the Behavior

Identifying when you are investing in a "spin" can be an interesting practice! One method that works for me is noticing if I feel especially emotional about a topic, I've probably invested in a way of looking at it.

There's a skill to changing your behavior, and over time you will be able to catch yourself closer and closer to the moment of actually doing it, until you are able to feel that you are *about* to do "that thing" and then stop yourself before you actually do.

This poem by Portia Nelson vividly describes this process of behavioral change:

Autobiography in Five Short Chapters

Chapter One

I walk down the street.

There is a deep hole in the sidewalk.

I fall in.

I am lost...I am helpless.

It isn't my fault.

It takes me forever to find a way out.

Chapter Two

I walk down the same street.

> There is a deep hole in the sidewalk.

> I pretend I don't see it.

> I fall in again.

I can't believe I am in this same place.

> > But, it isn't my fault.

It still takes a long time to get out.

Chapter Three

I walk down the same street.

There is a deep hole in the sidewalk.

I see it is there.

> I still fall in...it's a habit...but,

> > my eyes are open.

> > I know where I am.

It is *my* fault.

I get out immediately.

Chapter Four

I walk down the same street.

> There is a deep hole in the sidewalk.

> I walk around it.

Chapter Five

I walk down another street.[25]

Step Two: Take Ten Deep Breaths and Reset

Ana has founded her entire system of yoga on relentless, dedicated expansion of our breath capacity. Breath is the first of the four pillars of Forrest Yoga. In many ways, I feel that my biggest job is to teach my students to breathe better. Breathing well is at the heart of a good relationship with your body. The breath is a place of magic, where change is always present. The breath is so sensitive that it's affected by even just talking or writing about it. The breath is the key and the portal between your conscious self and your unconscious self. It is the way we switch modes from human animal to human spirit.

I also teach my students to explore the language of feeling inward *through* the breath. The breath is how we connect inward. We often try to think about our somatic and emotional experiences, but thinking takes us out of feeling. Our habitual behaviors have very much to do with our habitual ways of feeling. So if we want to track these in order to change our speech and behaviors, we must stay in feeling. To stay in feeling, stay connected to breath.

When people are not educated in how to breathe, when they hear "take a deep breath" they generally do something unhelpful: they inhale *fast* (fast is not deep—deep means long and slow), then they kinda *hold* their breath, and then they let it out in a big sigh.

The big sigh might be helpful, but the other two actions are decidedly *not*. Inhaling fast, and through the mouth, is what we do involuntarily when we are surprised or frightened (there's a name for this: a gasp). Holding the breath is something we do to try to manage tension, even though it has the exact opposite effect.

In Forrest Yoga, a "deep breath" means something very specific. I'll teach you.

Do this now:

1. Sit up tall.

2. Put your hands on your ribs wherever you can reach them.

3. Inhale slowly, through your nose, and press your ribs into your hands.

4. Exhale slowly, through your nose, and at the end of the exhale, pull your lower belly back toward your spine.

This is the beginning of deep breathing. Extend your inhale to last five seconds. Extend your exhale to match.

There's another aspect of deep breathing, called *ujjayii*. I'll describe it here, but it's better taught in person or through a visual demo. Please visit http://www.newharbinger.com/43430 to view an instructional video on this aspect of the Formula for Change (see the Resource Guide).

Ujjayi is a Sanskrit word that means "breath of victory" or Victorious Breath. I love this name, because armed with your breath, you will surely prevail over the obstacles before you in the great journey of your life.

Ujjayi also helps with deep breathing because it slows down the rate at which the air enters the lungs.

To create ujjayi:

1. Breathe out through your mouth, making a whisper sound at the back of your throat, like "haaaaaaaah"—that's the ujjayi sound.

2. Inhale through your mouth, again making that sound at the back of your throat.

3. Repeat.

4. Seal your lips and breathe out through your nose, still making that sound at the back of your throat.

5. Inhale through your mouth, making that sound at the back of your throat.

6. Repeat.

7. Now seal your lips again and breathe out through your nose, continuing to make that ujjayi sound.

8. Keeping your lips sealed, breathe in, still making the ujjayi sound.

9. Continue, listening to the sound of your breath. Notice that its sound is mostly the same on the inhale and the exhale, and that the length of the inhale and the exhale are the same.

Put ujjayi together with deep breathing, and now you have a breath that will change you and grow your breath capacity. Take *ten* of them now! At first you might feel a little dizzy—that's okay! Your entire body will quickly adjust to being fed more nourishing breath. When you change the way you breathe, you alter your physical state, which will affect how you feel. Ten deep breaths will intervene when you are about to make a judgment—good or bad!—and put you into a more intelligent state, accessing the wisdom of your body and all the feelings it contains. From there, you can make better decisions and experience better outcomes.

Step Three: Reward Yourself Lavishly for Catching the Behavior

Now that you've taken ten deep breaths, you're ready for the next step. This one is perhaps the most important. You've caught yourself thinking your old self-mutilating thought: *My belly is so flabby; I'm so ugly!*

It's tempting to beat ourselves up for doing the same old thing that we *know* isn't helpful.

Do not punish yourself! This will just more deeply entrench the behavior, and now you'll be caught up in an entirely *new* layer of behavior that you'll want to modify—self-recrimination. Self-recrimination is never helpful; regret, however, can be very educational.

Instead of punishing yourself, congratulate yourself. Just make sure you don't congratulate yourself with an addictive behavior. A congratulatory act may be just a simple internal shift toward compassion for yourself and your own suffering. It might be talking to a friend about the thoughts and emotions that are hurting you. It might be connecting with a person you really care about, going for a walk, or reading a book for ten minutes. What will ease the tension and put you into a state of kindness for yourself and your own suffering? What do you need to help yourself? Rewarding yourself will speed up the process of repatterning a new neurological response to your own thoughts, feelings, and behaviors. The body and the spirit respond to kindness and positivity.

Step Four: Take One Step Toward Healing

After congratulating yourself, you might consider what would be a step toward healing. (Sometimes the congratulations *is* that step.)

A step toward healing might be giving up dieting. It might be buying clothes that you love to wear on your body in its current manifestation. It might be giving away your scale. It might be unsubscribing from social media accounts that send you into a "things are so horrible" spiral. If you find yourself dealing with an injury, and you are having a hard time finding the "hidden potential," spend time meditating on that and sending compassionate energy *to* your injury. Talk to your injury. Ask what it wants you to learn and what it needs to feel better. If you're ill, take some of the same steps. If you're wrangling with aging, get honest with yourself about why it's bothering you. Are there things you've left undone that are calling for completion? Is the increasingly visible specter of death causing you to question your life? Talking to your body in this way isn't crazy. We talk to our bodies all the time—it's just that usually those conversations aren't constructive. These new kinds of conversations with the body engage its wisdom in a compassionate way.

To find out what the healing step is for you, you might need to meditate on that general question. Or journal. Or go for a walk to think about it. Engaging the body in the very process of discovery is a wise and potent choice.

Outwit the Spin Doctor

Knowing that we're going to spin a situation—because, hey, it's the human thing to do—we can prepare. It's useful to consider in advance some thoughts, situations, or experiences that cause spin. A spin trigger might be a social occasion with food. Or seeing someone who makes you feel bad about yourself, because they embody the things that you *think* they have and want. Or seeing yourself in a photo.

Follow these steps to help outwit your spin doctor, and prepare to be the best version of yourself under suboptimal circumstances. Title your page "Outwitting My Spin Doctor."

1. In your journal, list your current top three triggers.

2. What is the thought or the feeling that usually happens immediately afterward? What is the spin? Write these down.

3. Now, what are some different thoughts that you could choose to think? Write them down. They will feel awkward and contrived, but that's just change—like writing your name with your other hand.

4. Finally, who can you enlist and count on to give you a different perspective when your spin doctor is being cruel? Think of people whose perspective you trust, people you know have your best interests at heart. Write their names down somewhere, or put them in a special group in your phone so that when you forget, because you're caught up in the middle of a spin, you remember who they are. These are people I want you to form an alliance with—people you can call up when you need a fresh outlook. People you can rely on to pump you up, so to speak. I have this agreement with my friend Ruby. Sometimes I need a "general" pumping up. Sometimes it's specific. Either way, I *know* that I can count on her to come through when I'm in a time of need.

Like bragging, the pump-you-up aspect of a friendship can be a very healing agreement between women. We've been taught to compete, so having a friend you know will shine back at you the best about you when you are unable to see it for yourself does wonders for the heart and for the bonds between women in the past, present, and future.

Now, dear reader, you have made it to the halfway point in our journey together! Congratulations! This lesson about spin and change may be the real key you need to alter your relationship with all of the previous topics: happiness, competition, comparison, judgment, envy, and perfectionism. Look back over the prior lessons, if need be, with an eye for how you can tell yourself a different, inspiring, and increasingly truthful story about the circumstances of your life.

The big takeaway is this: we're empowered to make choices about our life conditions and events, and what and how we think about them. This is a huge mind-set shift, and your brain might need to be fed to support it—literally! We may not get to choose fundamental circumstances—our family of origin, our face and body, our innate gifts and talents—but we *can* choose how we respond to it all.

Real change is the road less traveled. Most prefer to maintain the status quo; it feels (deceptively) easier. The path is well worn. But if you'd like to change, you now have so many new, clear-sighted outlooks at your disposal for you to craft a life filled with feelings and experiences that you *and* your body like. Good for you! Ready to continue down that path with lots of exciting scenery?

Change starts with how you think about yourself and the world. But it is your body that *participates concretely* in the material world. To really connect the two—mind and body—we have to take care of the body. The next lesson really dives into what it means to be embodied. As we'll discover, while embodiment poses its own challenges, it's my sincere hope that by addressing the wounds held in the body we'll start to lay the groundwork for honestly healing them. Healing of all varieties is a natural process that we can access through an inner awareness of the body, and down this road lies freedom. How exciting! Onward!

Reclaim Your Body as Safe; Call Your Spirit Home

I developed early and attracted unwanted sexual attention. As a child in a woman's body, I didn't comprehend exactly what was happening, but I understood enough to know it was because of my body. As a result, I felt exceedingly *unsafe* in it. I blamed my body for the danger I sensed.

It's hard to overstate how often women feel menaced—and actually *are*. Our bodies endanger us; we're at risk for simply inhabiting a female body. So living within our body—that is, embodied—can feel treacherous, threatening our physical, emotional, and spiritual survival. Feeling unsafe in our body also can lead to feeling *fundamentally insecure being our authentic selves,* so disembodiment becomes a strategy for safety. As a girl I wrote in my journal: "I maintain a strained distance from my body." Though I didn't yet know what to call it, young Erica began disembodying.

I am a survivor of childhood sexual assault, and my wish to escape my body motivated me to be thin. If I lost weight, parts I identified as culpable for unwanted sexual desire and objectification would shrink. Smaller breasts, smaller hips, no ass, and for sure nothing that *jiggled* or *puckered:* this was an insurance policy against the unpredictability and potential danger of how others reacted to my female form. When I was thin, I figured, I could simply disappear. When it was shrouded in the invisibility of thinness, people couldn't objectify my body. I'd be safe, my humanity restored, and I could become a whole person with real assets to offer besides boobs and hips and ass. Through annihilating my female body I would become a valid, recognized, and viable human.

Being a woman is dangerous. One out of every six women in the United States will become the victim of an attempted or completed rape in her lifetime. Permissive attitudes toward rape have deep roots in Western society. In medieval France, the municipal authorities all but decriminalized it in cases where the victims were women of the lower class. In fourteenth-century Venice, the rape of an unmarried proletariat woman rarely called for more than a slap on the wrist, even in the frequent case when it involved group assault.[26] In the 1600s England's Chief Justice Matthew Hale warned that rape "is an accusation easily to be made and hard to be proved, and harder to be defended against the party accused." Judges in the US read the so-called Hale warning to juries until the 1980s.[27] Despite overwhelming evidence that women submit very few false rape accusations (in the low single digits), the Hale warning encouraged the public, and juries, to not believe rape victims' accusations, thus discouraging them from coming forward, and thereby perpetuating dismissive attitudes toward rape. In other words: rape culture. Our ancestral memory of institutionalized violence against women is real; it lives on in our bodies.

Our ancestral memory of institutionalized violence against women is real; it lives on in our bodies.

Some women starve and shrink to make themselves safe. Some women become fat to make themselves safe. The objective is the same—to disappear as a sexually attractive female and thereby acquire the protection of invisibility.

But it just doesn't work out like that. Deleting one part diminishes the whole. Erasure is inherently violent, and in harming our bodies, we also wound our spirits.

Imagine if you couldn't come home daily to a safe, welcoming environment. This is the way your spirit feels when you're disembodied: exiled from the only home it will ever have. It should break your heart just to consider this! This is *you* we're talking about, after all!

People describe a spiritless experience in terms that sound a lot like depression. Life loses its luster. Things that used to bring joy no longer do. Every day feels like a chore. Something ineffable and precious is slowly draining away from your body. You're not sure what you're doing with your life. These are the signs that your spirit is suffering.

You're not meant to be invisible. Shrinking the body and shrinking *within* the body is a way of being "less than." It's submission to a society that creates dangerous hierarchies. Disobey! Your spirit is meant to inhabit your body fully, and you're meant to learn to be brave enough to live in the world completely and embodied within your inherently fragile, flawed human form. This is how we learn compassion for our bodies and the beings within them, and that's what this lesson is all about. Yes, the world can be cruel, and it might also be an unsafe place, yet we can make our bodies a safe harbor for our spirits and learn to trust ourselves again. Embodiment is the way. Knowledge liberates, and just understanding a pattern starts to drain its power.

Let's look at some of the social factors that cause disembodiment—the first step in starting to loosen their hold on us.

THE CAUSES OF OBJECTIFICATION AND DISEMBODIMENT

The simple truth is, objectification leads to disembodiment.

The laws of the universe function on energy exchanges. For example: offer a prayer, receive a blessing. In this world of "this for that" we've learned to use our bodies as hard currency, or the object with which we'll strike a deal. In this act, we simultaneously overidentify (it's the thing of top value!) and disconnect from our bodies (objectification hurts!). Instead of existing rightfully as a sentient organism, the body becomes an unfeeling thing to trade. This is the process of objectification. But you are a human *being,* not a human *doing.* Your journey as an evolving soul requires you to remember this, and to protect your body.

We subjugate the body primarily though work and physical labor, fueling our own disconnect. Silvia Federici tells us that the German philosopher, economist, historian, and political theorist Karl Marx "sees the alienation from the body as a distinguishing trait of the capitalist work-relation. By transforming labor into a commodity, capitalism causes workers to submit their activity to an external order over which they have no control and cannot identify with. Thus, the labor process becomes a ground of self-estrangement."[28]

Like it or not, living in a capitalist society, we're enmeshed in value propositions encouraging us to disembody. Women, bound to our female bodies, experience three main pressures: desirability, reproductive capacity, and physical labor. It's as if we've been chopped up into pieces, with each one measured, and bearing a price tag. Our faces. Our wombs. Our hands. What's a gal to do? To free ourselves from damaging mind-sets, and to bring ourselves back to our rightful *embodied state,* we need to know how these mind-sets work, then watch how we bring them to life though talk and behavior. Only then can we make more empowered choices to disrupt these social patterns and transform lives.

The Value of a Beautiful Body (Face Included!)

When we evaluate the body for its beauty, we are objectifying it, and that objectification contributes to our disembodiment. In our primarily hetero-normative world we've been indoctrinated that our body's value resides in its desirability to a man, its beauty and sexual appeal. We conflate love and desire. We want to be loved; we think desire will lead there.

If you want to become more desirable, the body's beauty and desirability are a (small) aspect. From my observations, what men—and, honestly, just *people*—find attractive is a person who is happy, confident, and healthy, and who is sensual because she feels good in her own skin. Confidence is generated through experiencing positive outcomes. People react well to your looks, and this creates "looks" confidence. When people enjoy talking to you, this creates "great conversationalist" confidence. Some of us have confidence generated from our wardrobe. That's "clothes" confidence or "style" confidence. These are just a few aspects of self-confidence. Hating your body simply gets in the way.

What do you feel confident about in your life? Get out your journal and make a list! Title your page "Confidence Log" and follow the prompts.

- I feel confident about…

- I feel confident when I…

- I am confident that I can…

If confidence and desirability go hand in hand, it's important to know what makes you desirable. If you're not sure, check in with some of your closest friends. You can ask them: *What do you like and appreciate most about me? What makes you want to spend time with me?* Based on their responses, you'll have clues to where you can build your confidence. One of my clients was shocked to find out that her friends loved her generosity and her sense of humor. She had no clue this was the case! In possession of this new information, she began to paint a fresh picture of her desirability, and this altered her sense of self and thus her self-confidence.

Who are the top three people in your life you could go to for an honest reflection about what makes them want to spend time with and around you? List them in your journal. Do this now! Then make a date to interview them about yourself and ask the questions you just explored in your Confidence Log. Tell them you're trying to gain a better understanding of yourself so that you can grow as a person. Good friends will want to help you with this.

Also consider what you're good at. Skills are part of your assets. We generate self-confidence based on the experience of doing things well and having positive outcomes. Confidence is built on evidence that *you can.* Don't concern yourself with the question of talent versus acquired skill; let's focus on the idea that you can gain competency in whatever area you choose. What would you *like* to be good at, and why? These are some small but powerful questions to disrupt the standard, socially generated desirability metric. When you value deeper attributes within yourself and generate confidence in those, it realigns for others what is desirable about you.

In your journal, follow these prompts. Title your page "Skills Log."

1. What do you already feel like you're good at? List at least three things.

2. What are things you would *like* to be good at? Again, list at least three. (Why three? This is where you start to have flexibility, and the beginnings of freedom. One—you are a slave. Two—you have a dilemma. Three—you start to be free!)

3. Why would you like to be good at these things? How would that alter your sense of self?

4. Who would you be if you were good at this?

5. What would you be able to do in the world if you were good at this?

Ponder also what you especially like about yourself, regardless of whether other people see, recognize, or value those attributes. Buried treasure is still treasure. Ironically, shifting the value equation away from the body and onto personal attributes creates a more beautiful being, body included.

The Maternal Body's Value

When we evaluate the worth of the body solely for its ability to make another human, this can also exile the person within. The key admirable attribute of the mother is self-sacrifice. Disembodiment strikes again! Mothers literally sacrifice their body for the birth of a child. Sometimes fatally so.

When people feel confined by their sex, it crushes the spirit.

What about your own mother? Did she *really want* to be a mother? Maybe she didn't, but motherhood was one of few options available to her at the time. When people feel confined by their sex, it crushes the spirit.

How did having children affect *your* mother? Was she the person she most wanted to be? Did she live the life she most yearned for? She may have, and if so, that is terrific news.

Modern society *still* views women who can't procreate as "less valuable" and women who *won't* procreate as aberrations. Why?

Some answers from the past persist today. The very beginnings of our expatriation from our female bodies began with the witch hunts, fomented in Europe, then exported worldwide. The witch hunts are practically absent from our historical record, but they were a massive genocide, mostly uninvestigated and undocumented because women didn't have a voice. It's nearly impossible to estimate the number of women murdered in the witch hunts, for three main reasons: (1) historians rarely agree on the dates of the beginning and the end of the practice; (2) the victims, in Europe, were mostly undocumented peasant women; and (3) the very point of the witch hunts was to *erase* a population, their views, and collective knowledge. That's what genocides do. Estimates suggest that between 1450 and 1880, anywhere from fifty thousand to nine million women were murdered.

The witch hunts had a huge impact on our collective psyche and memory, even if, despite ample modern research and historical recovery, most historians tend to view it as folklore.

The witch hunts criminalized women's authority over their reproductive capacities, expropriated women from their bodies, transformed maternity into mandatory labor, and systematically erased healthy, collective female memory. Our bodies became objects. *The witch hunts forced us into disembodiment.* Previously normal activities, customs, and knowledge in the areas of herbalism and midwifery became forbidden to women. Women could be burned at the stake for any contraceptive initiative,

The witch hunts are the genesis of our body problems.

because it was viewed as the product of demonic perversion.[29] Women's bodies and reproductive capacities became the property of the state, quite literally.

Because our bodies were the site of two extremely valuable commodity creations—labor and therefore money—our foremothers were indoctrinated that their most basic and *compulsory* life work was to bear children. Enforced through torture and execution, this mindset was cemented so powerfully that even today it creates an inclination to value women based on the essential nature of our bodies, and *specifically* on our bodies' beauty, youth, and concomitant signs of childbearing potential. Even though today our population is steadily growing—straining the planet's capacity to support all of us sustainably—and there's an abundance of people to work, and we have plenty of food, the terror experienced centuries ago still ensures ongoing and enduring compliance.

For most women, having a child is a beautiful experience. But that's not all that's valuable about you as a woman. If you don't use your body for its maternal value (or even if you do, or have), what other goods and services do you have to offer the world? (Yes, in capitalism, a child is a product—just think of its Social Security number as its bar code!)

Review your Skills Log from the previous section and build on it. Is there anything else you'd like to add?

What other gifts come from having a female body? One of my teachers, Alison Armstrong, defines innate talents that originate from being female as *feminine forms of power.* The feminine works though invisible means and creates where once there was nothing. This is why having babies is so awe-inspiring. Our bodies have an empty space in which another body (a child) can be created. This is pure magic. But this isn't our only form of power. What else do you uniquely bring into an empty space? When

The body remembers, even if the conscious mind does not.

you enter the room, what comes with you? What else do you, uniquely, create out of nothing?

I've found that some of the innate gifts that I bring are grounded-ness, calm, insight, understanding, and wisdom. My friends call me, or want to spend time with me, when they want a dose of these elements, which are invisible to the eye. Despite their unseen nature, they effect change in the people around me. After a particularly deep yoga class, one of my students said to me, with excitement, "When you teach yoga, I *understand* so much more!" I laughed because, well, this is one of my gifts to the world: understanding. It's why I wanted to write this book.

Bringing these felt qualities into existence from where once there was nothing is a kind of birthing. It's using the maternal female body for other, spiritual means. Because these characteristics don't exist in the world until you embody them. Understanding, for instance, is simply a nice idea until it is *experienced,* which means *the body feels it.* Can you see this? Your body is the vessel through which all your most valuable assets manifest. There is no other way to go about it.

What are your forms of feminine power? You'll see their little foot-prints in the way they create a change in the people around you—how they relate to you and value you—and in what kinds of people you attract. Shifting the focus from what the body can do to what and who you can be in your body will help you become more embodied.

Really ponder this, and journal on it! Title your page "My Feminine Forms of Power." When I coach my yoga business clients, I ask them this power-ful question: *What, above all, do you want your students to learn from you?* This is a way of asking them what is most important for them to manifest and embody. For you, because you probably aren't a yoga teacher, you can consider what feelings are the most important to you—for yourself, and for the people around you to experience. Use these as clues to what your own forms of feminine power are.

The Machine Body

Prior to the Industrial Revolution, the body was magical. After that transformative change to society, the body became a machine. When the body is a machine, it tends to disembody us.

"The machine body" developed along with mechanical philosophy, an understanding of the universe as subject to predetermined laws, which means everything is orderly and predictable as a clock. Silvia Federici notes that in René Descartes' *Treatise on Man* (1631), the father of modern Western philosophy insists that "this machine" (as he persistently calls the body) is just an automaton, and its death is no more to be mourned than the breaking of a tool.[30] What a desolate view!

The very *first* invention of mechanical philosophy was its deconstruction of the human body. Its constitutive elements—from the circulation of the blood to the dynamics of speech, from the effects of sensations to voluntary and involuntary motions—were taken apart and classified in all their components and possibilities.[31] The heart was viewed as just a spring; the musculoskeletal system, pulleys and strings. Cartesian philosophy saw the mind and body as separate, created not as an organic being imbued with its own intelligence, but as a simple, stupid, unfeeling, machine.

The body was quite literally dehumanized by this belief. What died along with its humanity was its capacity as a receptacle for magical powers connected with nature. The death of the body's whims and needs was necessary to create a disciplined and obedient work force. Magic cannot be neatly tamed and made to labor at prescribed hours. Magic is unruly! To make the body labor like a machine—in modern life, for example, sitting at a desk or working on an assembly line for eight to ten hours a day—there simply *cannot* be space for the body to have its own organic needs.

The "body is a machine" mind-set shows up so many places: medicine, work expectations, and weight loss, for example. It shows up in the idea of "calories in, calories out"—wherein feeding the body is equivalent to fueling, as all calories are considered equal and therefore utilized and burned equally. In Gary Taubes' *Why We Get Fat: And What to Do About It,* he painstakingly dismantles the calories in/calories out model, showing with science that the metabolism is affected by hormones, genetics, a prior history of malnutrition and starvation for the person *or their mother,* and a history of weight loss.[32] What we eat and how it shows up on the body isn't merely the result of simple math. Also, in Taubes' research he considers *female* bodies. I've found that, so often, when it comes to the notion of calories in/calories out, men cite only themselves and then wonder why women have such a hard time with this orderly, logical notion. It's as if they assume women's bodies function exactly like theirs! But they don't. First, there's that second pesky X chromosome. Then there is the matter of cyclical hormones. A body bathed in estrogen and progesterone functions differently from one washed in testosterone.

Anyway, were it true that the body's just a simple machine, disciplining wouldn't be necessary. Machines don't need self-restraint! Animals do. Most people view being called an animal an insult. I invite you to reconsider our place in the fabric of being and view our bodies as part of a beautiful animal kingdom. Every body is magical, with the capacity for its own intelligence, consciousness, and memory. Do *you* know how to heal? *No.* The body does. Do you know how to make a baby? *No.* Do you know how to grow hair, fingernails, and skin? *No.* The body does. How? This is exactly the magic and the genius of the body. When we eradicate the Cartesian declaration that the body is a machine, an object solely useful for its beauty, reproductive abilities, and capacity to work, we restore our innate dignity, humanity, and *fundamental sacredness.* While reinstating our humanity, we can come home to the body and live in it embodied as we've always been meant to.

Tally the various ways you treat your body as if it were a machine. Do you push it for long hours at work, perhaps confined to a desk chair? Do you expect it to continue, even if you're sick or injured? Do you provide it with enough sunlight, fresh air, nutritious food, play, movement, and rest, taking care of it like an animal (or plant!) you really care about?

In the United States, mostly we don't rest enough. One of the great powers of the body is its capacity to heal, and most regeneration occurs while we sleep. Ancient societies once worshipped the bear, who was an avatar for the Great Mother. The magical power of the bear is, in addition to her fierce mothering, her capacity to heal. During the time that bears rest (hibernate), they repair. Part of the feminine power of the human body is rest, repair, and regeneration. To counter how deeply you've been indoctrinated in your value measured through work, take stock of how well you rest. Give yourself permission to sleep. Give yourself time to dream. Give yourself time to heal, restore, and regenerate. These are some of the great powers of the body when we allow it. When we actually take real care of the body, it promotes our own embodiment.

Disembodiment Costs You Your Spirit

Mechanization objectifies the body. Without practices that encourage embodiment—giving the body space to move, feeding it well, allowing it time to rest, regenerate, and heal—it's far easier to be cruel to the body. We may begin to deny feeling pain—or feeling anything at all, for that matter. Once disembodied, we'll *also* use our disembodiment to manage self-inflicted suffering. In a cruel cycle of self-abandonment, we further the objectification.

Tiny acts of violence become normalized. We don't eat. We don't sleep. We work too hard and move too little. We touch ourselves in ways that could never be described as kind. Poke. Prod. Pinch. Cut. We take pain pills and have surgery, never *truly* addressing the sources of our pain on their own terms, not once *really* addressing our bodies in ways that will truly help and repair them. We continue to deprive the body, because, hey, it's just an object. Consequently, our spirit withers. Though social pressures set the stage, we mostly do this to ourselves.

What a dark road! Where is the path back to the light? If you've read this far, you probably know by now that the body is the path. It's quite circular. The body is the beginning; it is the end. It's the alpha; it's the omega. One of my teachers, Matthew Sanford, observes, "I have never seen anyone truly become more aware of his or her body without also becoming more compassionate."[33] Knowing the body is the road home.

Knowing the body is the road home.

EMBODIMENT'S CHALLENGE: FEELING HURTS! (AT FIRST)

All of the elements of a human being are contained within one vessel: the body. Our minds are capable of taking us into the past and future, but the body exists only now. Therefore, for us to be truly embodied, all parts of us must be here now. I noted in the introduction that *embodiment* means integrating all the aspects of ourself in our body and fully experiencing the feelings of living from within our body. Only when we are truly here, now, can we access the body's complete intelligence and wisdom.

When we're smarter, we make better decisions and experience better outcomes. This is a great reward for embodiment!

The primary challenge to embodiment is pain—physical, emotional, intellectual, and spiritual. The trouble with full embodiment is that *everything hurts!* At least at first. Then it gets better, and everything is *everything.*

Bodies Hurt

When we make a commitment to living embodied, it means that we can no longer use disembodiment as a strategy for managing our physical pain. Darn.

Living with chronic pain can make us unrecognizable to ourselves. A client I've been working with for a number of years now came to me because, in his words, "his body was falling apart." He couldn't hold a coffee cup. His neck had been broken. He'd had surgery on both shoulders. He experienced sciatica. The pain's constant presence was

Embodiment makes us smarter.

making him irritable, ornery, and unpleasant to be around. Together we reduced his physical pain level considerably, and his yoga practice became a source of pain relief and even immense physical pleasure. He noticed he became much more pleasant and resilient to stress, and that he liked himself more as a result. He became recognizable to himself again. Once out from under the daily, debilitating effects of chronic pain, he's better able to review his life, to look at where he is going and what he wants next. When chronic pain is your daily crucible, it's harder to do this meta work.

His story is extreme, but not uncommon. We're all living with nagging discomforts big and small. When ignored for years, aches and pains gain strength, becoming actual injury or illness. The energy you use managing pain is energy you could be using to live your life in a far more satisfying way.

Small failures to manage physical pain escalate and can balloon out of control, turning into an emergency. The current opioid addiction crisis in the US is ample evidence of where these failures can lead (not to mention the emerging fact that these lucrative drugs were aggressively promoted as nonaddictive). Substance abuse and addiction of all kinds help mask our most fundamental pain while contributing to the overall problem, further taxing the body's resources. Above all, reliance on pain medications obstructs access to the primary avenue to self-knowledge: the physical.

What a Faustian bargain! Embodiment is painful. But the way home to the body is to address the pain in the body. The good news is, once you address the pain, you have the possibility of freeing it up. Once you release the pain, your spirit has a happier home to abide within. Abandon the fantasy disembodiment permits and get real, and you're on the road to freedom.

Becoming embodied can feel like arriving home to a house on fire.

To address the body's pain, you must have a non-outcome-oriented movement practice. This practice is a place where you can explore what your body is and how it feels. Yoga is quite well suited for this, but you might select something like tai chi, qigong, dancing, walking, swimming, or running, for example. It's not about fitness or accomplishment. It's about movement exploration. It needs to be a full-bodied movement practice. For instance, archery (one of my favorites!) doesn't count because that's mostly about isolating and refining small, generally static motions. Choose something that allows you time and space to just be and feel while moving fully. *You must move your body, in whatever way you are able to.*

In my private practice in New York City, I work with people who cannot move freely due to age or affliction. We find how they *can* move and work there. There is *always* something you can do. One of my students recounted being in a restorative yoga-teacher training, and working with a man who uses a wheelchair. For him, the experience of relaxing his arms in a supported posture drained away the pain, tension, and backlogged emotion caught up in using his arms for literally everything.

Movement, and sometimes stillness, is key to addressing the body's pain, freeing it up, and draining it away. Find out what you can do, every day. Develop a repertoire. I don't *want* to do yoga every day. Sometimes I want to swim. Sometimes I go for a long walk. Sometimes I lift some weights.

It seems so simple, but it's not.

You might wonder *how can I know which is needed?* The intuitive and discerning process of figuring it out relies on already having a relationship with the body. To make decisions about what the body needs, you cannot simply fall back on notions that rely on "the body as a machine." You cannot be seduced by the body-alienating, autonomy-robbing idea that you can't really know anything about the body without scientific evidence. To become open to and empowered by the information you receive from your own body requires that you invest in a relationship with that body. It's a circular process. You have to start somewhere! Movement is medicine. Find yours and use it daily. Explore how you feel and what seems to work for you, and why.

Emotions Hurt; Thoughts Hurt Too

After addressing our physical pain, we will probably slam into the full force of our emotions and dark, painful thoughts. But when we become embodied, we agree to feel it. *All of it.*

Pema Chödrön notes how the Buddhist master Trungpa Rinpoche describes emotion: as a combination of self-existing energy and thoughts.[34] The energy of the emotions exists in our bodies. The thoughts take place in the "intellectual" aspect of our minds. Emotions cannot proliferate without our internal conversations.[35] In other words, it's the stories (thoughts) we tell ourselves about the energies we feel in our bodies that cause our emotions to stick around.

The process goes like this.

1. You have an emotion or a feeling.

2. You have a thought about that emotion or feeling.

3. The thought creates another feeling.

4. Often you create an opinion (thoughts) about it all (you little spin doctor, you!).

5. This creates another feeling.

6. And you keep spiraling like this until you've created a real tangle for yourself!

7. All of this thinking keeps the painful emotions alive! *Ouch!*

But you can intervene at any moment. How? By refusing to think. By *just feeling.* Sounds simple enough, right?

Until you try it—and find that thoughts and emotions stick to each other so strongly, it can be challenging to disentangle them. Is it a thought? Is it a feeling? Discerning is part of the skill in getting them to stop hurting so much. Often our thoughts are even more harmful than the emotions! If you look back at lessons 1 through 4, you'll see that they're all about the kinds of thoughts that hurt us. If you've done the exercises in those chapters, you've already done much work in this area. (Congratulations!)

When you experience something upsetting and have a reaction to it, try asking yourself *What is the emotion I am experiencing,* and *What thoughts am I having about my emotions?* An even more powerful question, posed to me by my massage therapist, is *What if this was pleasurable?* Can you change the experiences you perceive of as painful into pleasure? Instead of resisting, he suggested, give your consent for all that you encounter while feeling. It is, after all, our resistance that creates the painful friction.

Don't struggle! Surrender! Why?

> [In] Buddhism it is said that wisdom is inherent in emotions. When we struggle against our energy we reject the source of wisdom. Anger without the fixation is none other than clear-seeing wisdom. Pride without fixation is experienced as equanimity. The energy of passion when it's free of grasping is wisdom that sees all angles.[36]

Staying with our emotions (which are energies within the body) and finding their very core, we become *embodied.* We're smartest when we're embodied. We make better, faster decisions, behave more authentically, and experience outcomes based on the truth of our experiences. These are great benefits.

I learned these concepts while using the body in my yoga practice. The irony of writing about embodiment is that these words will get you only part of the way to embodiment. Why? The body doesn't speak English.

Embodied learning is especially powerful, leading to embodied knowledge. Since all parts of you exist in your body, to address the pain held in your emotional and intellectual body it's essential to address the body simultaneously. And, of course, embodiment is best taught in person (duh!). (I'd love to see you in my next workshop or retreat. Come to class when you are in New York City! Visit my website to see when the next workshop or retreat is happening.)

The body doesn't speak English.

But you can begin to work on this here and now. Here are two exercises.

- Go inside yourself. What emotions do you feel right now? Chances are you feel an emotional reaction to what you're reading. What is it? Where do you feel it in your body? Can you breathe into that area and feel your feelings as completely as you can? Try using ujjayii, taught in Lesson 4. (For a tutorial or review, revisit the video instruction at http://www .newharbinger.com/43430.) Study what changes when you begin to do that. Perhaps you're having thoughts, and a story you're already telling yourself about your feelings. Stop. Just breathe. Just feel. That's all. Sit with your emotions, and allow their purest wisdom to surface. *Allow your feelings to* just be *without creating any narrative.*

- I call this second exercise "Mood Modulation." First, observe your mood. Then use your movement practice *specifically* with the intent of shifting your mood. This acknowledges that when you are feeling an emotion, it lives in your body, and if you move your body, you can *create* a shift and actually generate a specific mood. How would you like to *feel?* What kind of movement can you do to put you in that specific mood? One of my New York fitness friends, Rupa Mehta, designed a book around this concept—how can you move and eat to affect your mood?[37] The ways that we move, especially in yoga, affect our nervous system and therefore can alter our moods in specific ways. Pretty cool!

Embodiment's Reward: Coming Home to the Magical Body

Objectifying the body, living disembodied—both of these mean living without your spirit. The witch hunts, the transition from feudalism to capitalism, and the Industrial Revolution drove a wedge between us and our bodies, and therefore between our bodies and our spirits.

Silvia Federici explains that in the Middle Ages, prior to the witch hunts, the body was believed to possess magical powers:

At the basis of magic was an animistic conception of nature that did not admit to any separation between matter and spirit, and thus imagined the cosmos as a *living organism,* populated by occult forces, where every element was in "sympathetic" relation with the rest. In this perspective, where nature was viewed as a universe of signs and signatures, marking invisible affinities that had to be deciphered…every element—herbs, plants, metals, and most of all the human body—hid virtues and powers peculiar to it.[38]

"Magic" could take any manner of forms, but the central theme is that it relied on chaotic forces of nature and defied mechanical (scientific) explanation. Examples of magic include mesmerism, soothsaying, necromancy, spiritualism, herbalism, astrological prediction, divination, and tarot readings. All precapitalist societies believed in the magic power of such pursuits. Recently we're seeing a resurrection of practices historically condemned as witchcraft. The revival of magical beliefs is possible today because it no longer represents a social threat to commerce. Federici notes: "Astrology…can be allowed to return, with the certainty that even the most devoted consumer of astral charts will automatically consult the watch before going to work."[39]

Within this environment, the ideas I'm sharing—that your body is part of the natural world, that you can trust it, that you can be safe in your body even if the outside world is unsafe, that it can be a source of wisdom otherwise unavailable to your intellect—can be voiced without the threat of condemnation as a witch, and without the specter of torture and execution. Hurrah!

In fact, you can now openly use "witch" as a proud and rebellious label. When one of my clients recounts what I've done for him, he tells people "She's a witch." I don't *encourage* this type of sales pitch, yet it's not an entirely inaccurate description of talents and skills I've discovered and cultivated only since being on a path of peace and acceptance with my body. These are parts of myself, in fact, that I consider more honest, real, and true than the kind of woman I was trying to become prior to discovering a path of living embodied.

You can reclaim your body as a safe home without self-identifying as a witch, or other vogue terms like shaman or goddess. Your body possesses information that escapes and even defies logic. This is magical. That's all you really need to know. Sometimes we define the magical occurrence of things we don't understand as a miracle. Embrace miracles and magic, and you'll begin to repair centuries of conditioning that divorced us from our female bodies.

The body is a part of nature, a part of the life force that exists in all things, a part of the divine. Humans are intrinsically magical. You are a miracle.

Simply described, magic is our ability to change, transform, or evolve. Where there was an acorn and now there is a tree? Magic. A body that creates a baby? Magic. Someone who brokers peace where once there was strife? Magic. *Creation of any kind is magical; it's the essence of change.* It's really that simple, not scary or inexplicable. Magic is everyday. The delusion that we're separate from the natural world is an invention to assuage our consciences over its destruction. We objectify the world we live in as mere material for our purposes, not as a manifestation of the divine life force. This mirrors our own self-objectification.

Changing the way you think is a kind of magic, because when you change the way you think, you change your view of the world; then the world appears different, and indeed it *is* different. Where once you hated yourself, now you love yourself. Magic. *How did you do it?* they all will ask. And it will be hard to say, exactly, because the story happened in your body.

Embrace miracles and magic, and you'll begin to repair centuries of conditioning that divorced us from our female bodies.

It might help you to consider the body as "bigger" than you. Let go a little from the need to know, control, or understand. Yield to the great mystery of life.

Acknowledging your body's divinity, magical capacities, and great unknown might help you relinquish some of the misplaced and erroneously conceived responsibility for all you perceive to be its failings. So much of life is out of our control. The body is magical, not logical. And that means it's not really under our control either. This might be a helpful or comforting thought when you try to discipline it via dieting or exercise. You're fighting a failing battle, so why not put down your weapons? Embrace your body as the divine, wild, incomprehensible thing it is, and perhaps that will take you down a new, more joyful path.

What does that look like? Some coaches feel that to truly, honestly live abundantly you *must* unleash and reclaim your wild, insatiable, feminine sexual energy. Use a jade egg. Take up sensual dance, pole dancing, or stripping. These are wonderful, feminine embodiment practices for which I don't possess expertise. You might try some of them. I don't think that these things are *necessary* for you to come home to your body. As a mandate, they might create a form of femininity that is aggressive and demanding.

Yield to the great mystery of life.

Each woman will have her own journey. Yoga is my wheelhouse. I think it's especially effective because of the way Ana Forrest taught me to use the breath. Breathing helps us stop thinking so much and instead gets us into feeling, where all the body's wisdom lives.

Each of us has her own curriculum of healing, transformation, and contribution. You have the right to go at your own pace and do only what works for you at the moment. Right now, it's a good start to open your awareness to your body as magical. Start there. Appreciate what is does for you every day. Your heart beats. Your hair grows. Your food gets digested. Amazing. It has survived trauma. It's still surviving all the daily cruelty we commit. What a miracle. Be amazed.

You don't have to view your body as magical to reclaim it as a safe home. You can take all the steps I've previously outlined, and already you will be on a path to embodiment, which will improve your quality of life. Making a simple, concrete, logical commitment to addressing your daily physical, emotional, and spiritual pain will go very far indeed to making your life better. Of what I've presented here, take what immediately resonates, and leave the rest. It will still be here for you when you are ready.

EXPLORE YOUR HOME'S PREFERENCES

In Forrest Yoga, my teacher Ana often teaches thematic classes entitled "Delight Your Spirit" or "Romancing the Spirit." Her idea is simple, in a way, but not easy. It's a summation of this chapter, really. Your spirit resides within your body. (Where else could it possibly be?) Violence makes the body an inhospitable home for the spirit. The way to invite your spirit home is to delight it, and to romance it. How? A good way to start is by taking care of the body, finding out what pleases the body and what feeds the heart. Pleasure, delight, joy—these are some of the nutrients for the spirit.

Do you know what your body likes? We'll spend time in the next chapter exploring this further, but for now, I want to introduce you to a survey of the senses. It's a meditation to help you begin to make friends with the body, through its avenue of experiencing the world: the five senses.

Do this now. Grab your journal and title the page "What Delights My Senses."

Answer these questions.

1.   What do you love the sight of?

2.   What do you love the smell of?

3.   What do you love the sound of?

4.   What do you love the taste of?

5.   What do you love the feeling of, on your skin?

Answer with as many items as you can. Remember—three is where you'll begin to experience freedom!

I'll start, with a few per category.

1.   *Sight:* My answer: The sparkle of wind rippling water. My cat's fur face. The art on my apartment walls. The view of the New York skyline at sunset. The sight of the moon from my window. The view of the sky through leaves, lying on my back in the grass.

2. *Smell:* My answer: Leaves fallen from trees. Bergamot. Boxwood trees in the summer. Baking bread. Coffee.

3. *Sound:* My answer: My friend Ruby's laughter. Trains on train tracks. Crows calling to one another. Robins looking for a mate in the spring. The music of J. S. Bach. Cicadas in July.

4. *Taste:* My answer: Rhubarb cake. Mountain pie. Russian Fluff casserole. Poached eggs. Homemade vanilla ice cream.

5. *Feel:* My answer: Swimming—water on my skin. My cat's fur under my hand. Snakes—their muscles and scales are *amazing!* The weight and warmth of a sheepskin coat. The feeling of wind. Sailing—sun, water, wind all together. The momentum of cresting a hill on horseback.

I know that these things are true, because making this list got me crying. I've learned that the sign my spirit is here, now, and experiencing this with me is tears. Things that are real, true, honest, and valuable bring tears to my eyes. Stay alert to what is the sign for you that truth is afoot.

Once you've made this list, find out how you can build more of these sensory experiences in your life. Please your body through its senses. You start to know and take care of your body from within. Knowing your body, spending time—these are first steps to making it a safe place for you again. Along the way, you can begin to call your spirit home.

We all have a right to feel safe within our own skin. I'm so sorry this isn't the experience of most women, and that we have to work so hard to get back this feeling of security and trust. Nevertheless, it needs to be done. This relationship, with your body, is the *most important* relationship of your life. It is the foundation of everything you can and will be, because everything—*everything!*—comes into existence *through* your body.

In this lesson, we've gone over the many materialist currencies of exchange we leverage through the body—beauty, maternity, labor— and explored alternative value propositions. We discovered how moving through the pain of embodiment leads you to a true understanding of your feelings. The reward of this gnarly work is coming home, not to just a basic domicile, but to a magical, wild, and wonderful habitat called your body. This is really coming home to your self. Looking ahead, we'll explore using your body as *the tool* through which you will discover all of your self.

The core practice of sensory exploration can become a daily ritual of connecting to your body. In the lessons ahead, we're going to investigate larger subjects, continuing to find out exactly what the body needs to support your embodiment, growing health, and mystical path of self-discovery and transformation. These are some of my *very favorite* topics. I'm looking forward to sharing them with you!

You dove down into the weeds. Now it's time to press up toward the light. Let's go!

Your Body and Beauty Are Unique

In my twenties and early thirties, I played the piano professionally. When a renowned musician from Cuba came to town—which was a big deal because of the embargo!—I was hired to play the after-concert house party.

I have long, thick, dark hair, and when I played the piano, to get it out of the way I'd arrange it into double French braids. At the party a man and a woman there fawned over my looks. "Oh, my god!" they exclaimed. "You look *exactly* like Frida Kahlo! If you went to Mexico with your hair like that, the people would stop in the street thinking that you were she!"

I had never heard of Frida Kahlo. They were aghast at my ignorance. They told me, "Frida is a great beauty and an artist of staggering importance!" How was it possible I'd never heard of her?

That night I told my mother about this experience. She shrugged, not as enthused as I was. "Yes," she said. "I've often thought that. But never mentioned it, because Frida's looks are not really...ideal."

I was shocked. My mother *knew* of this mysterious woman who was absolutely *revered* by a whole nation of people, yet did not see fit to mention the resemblance, and in fact withheld the knowledge, because...I didn't know why! Was my own mother telling me she thought I was ugly?

My feelings changed from shock into quiet questioning. I started to research Frida and her story. I studied photographs of her, with her bold uni-brow, her singular sartorial sensibilities, and her unflinching confrontations with self, death, love, life, conflict, art, and politics. What a formidable *human being!* Her beauty stemmed not just from her face and her body, but from the person she was, her suffering, and the way she transmuted it into distinctive art, beauty, and joy. Looking at her, considering her as a woman, my thoughts about my own looks and value started to shift.

Feminine can mean what you want it to. Be your own kind of woman.

I started to question my mother's standards of beauty that, unbeknownst to me, I had inherited. If other people thought that Frida was beautiful—and, beyond that, an important *contributor* to her cultural heritage—then maybe I could also be those things.

CYBERSPACE ROLE MODELS

An old friend says: *Everyone is unique. But that doesn't make them distinct.*

What does he mean by this? One thing is for sure—barring cloning, there will never be another human being with your exact genetic coding. You are unique.

We come into this life with a lottery of genetics and character. You might call this *first nature. Second nature* is who you become, though your own efforts, and what you earn in the world. Our bodies don't look the way they do through merit alone; it's primarily an accident of genetics, and then how we tend to ourselves. Bodies are first nature. Second nature is our true mark of distinction, our truest beauty revealed.

So much of Frida Kahlo's beauty emanates from her second nature.

Although human bodies are infinitely varied, the media shows us a very narrow representation. When depictions lack diversity, that shapes our ideas of what is "normal" and how we "should be." Seeing uniformity in the bodies of models leads us to believe that one body type is "normal," although nothing could be further from the truth.

Just look around! It's unusual to see identical body shapes and sizes in one place. Nature favors variety.

The media also shows a consistent beauty ideal through photo manipulation and touch-ups. Photographs are falsified constructions altered to meet artificial standards of symmetry and consistency.

Teaching yoga in New York City is a personal reality check. I see hundreds of different bodies every week. I wish everyone had this vantage point. It still strikes me how very different everyone is and how the dimensions of all those bodies are slightly—or extremely— different from each other. It's really quite astonishing when you think about it.

Second nature is our true mark of distinction, our truest beauty revealed.

Social media brought us a whole new category of people called "Instagram models"—and online filters can easily slim a waist or puff up a booty or make eyes bigger and rounder. Now others feel free to state bluntly and publicly their opinions about people's bodies, faces, and clothes, heightening their seeming importance.

The upshot is that online, women of all sizes, shapes, colors, ages, genders, and ability are taking charge of their own representations. And the world is responding. Followers, corporations, and mainstream advertising have taken note. An incredible diversity in role models is available to us now! Instead of being force-fed role models preapproved by an ad agency, you can choose your own.

One of my very favorite things to do on social media (Instagram, specifically) is following people of all kinds to curate a more real and diverse version of visual reality. Here are some of my favorite accounts in the vanguard of the body acceptance movement: establishing trends and shaping conversations:

@effyourbeautystandards: Started by plus-size model Tess Holliday, this inspirational account shows women of all sizes, shapes, and colors *rocking* their bodies, fashion, fitness, and lifestyle.

@iconaccidental: This account features a sixty-four-year-old Fordham professor sporting big sunglasses and stylish outfits in an urban setting. She's a silver fox!

@alleles: This account features prosthetic limbs, beautifully rendered as fashion, and gorgeous images of the people who wear and use them.

You can tailor your personal social media to rewrite the visual story mainstream media has told you! When you start to create space in your visual field for many different and glorious forms of beauty, this also gives your permission and stimulates *you* to reimagine yourself in your own true and authentic form.

Once you start to give your wounds a chance to heal by not poking them daily with soul-assaulting imagery, I also think that it's a good practice to follow some accounts that you find annoying, confronting, or even offensive. Why? It's great training in:

- Educating yourself about how others view and experience the world

- Getting strong and resilient in your own center

- Becoming more tolerant and open-minded

In today's world, we can also easily curate our social media to create echo chambers, such that we become indignant when people dare to disagree. Respectfully disagreeing is a skill we need to practice! Knowing what the opposition believes helps us prepare respectful, insightful counter-arguments. Annoying people are very educational. Keep a few "good" ones in your social media stream! They will continuously remind you to be more yourself.

Annoying people are very educational. Keep a few "good" ones in your social media stream!

KNOW THY SELF

When I started practicing yoga in New York City, people were talking a lot about "learning to love yourself." This confused me, because I didn't know what "my self" was anyway. Knowing your "self" and then doing the work of "learning to love your self" assumes from the outset that we know what and who we are. But mostly we don't. *Self* is such a huge concept. Where to begin? We feel overwhelmed by the task because we intrinsically understand the vastness of our being. *We are immeasurable inside.*

Yoga describes the concept of a human in terms of five "bodies"— or *koshas*—a Sanskrit word that translates roughly as "sheath." The idea is, each sheath nests within the other, like a sword in a scabbard. I like to visualize those Russian dolls, where when you open each one, another smaller one is nesting within.

It can be hard for us to make sense of the hidden worlds and invisible aspects of ourselves. This difficulty keeps us ensnared in the primary conflict of being alive: We are our bodies, but we are not our bodies. The *koshas* describe our parts unseen and help us understand them.

We are our bodies, but we are not our bodies.

The *Taittiriya Upanishad*, a sacred yogic text, describes the koshas:

Human beings consist of a material body built from the food they eat. Those who care for this body are nourished by the universe itself.

Inside this is another body made of life energy. It fills the physical body and takes its shape. Those who treat this vital force as divine experience excellent health and longevity because this energy is the source of physical life.

Within the vital force is yet another body, this one made of thought energy. It fills the two denser bodies and has the same shape. Those who understand and control the mental body are no longer afflicted by fear.

Deeper still lies another body comprised of intellect. It permeates the three denser bodies and assumes the same form. Those who establish their awareness here free themselves from unhealthy thoughts and actions, and develop the self-control necessary to achieve their goals.

Hidden inside it is yet a subtler body, composed of pure joy. It pervades the other bodies and shares the same shape. It is experienced as happiness, delight, and bliss.[40]

These "bodies" have unique names.

- The "food body"—the part of you that we all can see—is called *annamaya kosha*.

- The "energy body"—the part of you that keeps all of your vital functions running, like your breathing, your heart beating, your digestion moving—is called the *pranamaya kosha*.

- The "mind body"—the part of you that animates your senses of sight, sound, taste, touch, and seeing—is called the *manomaya kosha*.

- The "intellectual body"—the part of you that thinks, discerns, and possesses will—is called the *vijnanamaya kosha*.

- The "bliss body"—the part of you that is connected to everything and *is* all things— is called the *annandamaya kosha*. It observes all of the other functions free of praise or judgment.

These bodies constitute aspects of consciousness and different ways we experience the world. It's striking to see that, according to the yogic philosophy, the physical body comprises only one-fifth of a human being. This philosophy points out that we give so much weight and importance to a part of us that's so small relative to the other components identified by the yogic tradition!

As I've studied the concept of the *koshas* and applied it to myself, I've found it's a tremendously useful model for learning to know, take care of, and eventually love your self. This five-part model helps us to disassemble and organize the endeavor. What does each *kosha* need to be nourished? When you delve into yogic philosophy, discovering these answers is key to understanding the mysterious and magical being that is you. When you create a relationship with each facet, learn how to take care of each and every piece, then you have a thorough and comprehensive understanding of "your self"—*the self that belongs to you.* You're better prepared first to love yourself and then to ask and answer the important life questions *What are you? What are you here for?*

We got a head start on this self-discovery in Lesson 5 with the sensory exploration, which addresses how the mind *kosha* (the third one) permeates the body via your senses. In the rest of this lesson, we'll take a close look at how to take care of the materially manifest aspects of ourselves (our body and our energies), which are the first and second *koshas.* In the final lesson we'll examine how to take care of the remaining subtle and ethereal aspects of a human, contained in the fourth and fifth *koshas.*

YOUR MARK OF DISTINCTION

What makes a body—and therefore the human being within it— begin to stand out is the care you give to tending the one body you have stewardship over for this lifetime. When the body shines, it helps make *all* of you shine and helps you find your true work in the world. You gain distinction.

When the body is cared for, it creates an inner luminosity that's difficult to describe.

Thích Nhất Hạnh says, "If you can accept your body then you can see your body as home. You have to accept yourself as you are. This is a very important practice. As you practice building a home in yourself you become more and more beautiful."

True beauty emerges from bravely engaging with all of your life experiences.

Frida Kahlo's beauty was built on her deep engagement with her own traumatic injury, resultant sickness, and ongoing pain and disappointment. She learned *how* to take care of her body and the spirit within specifically *through* her own pain. Her beauty is distinctive.

To take care of this one, utterly unique body you've been given for this life time, to care for it so thoroughly and honestly that the spirit begins to radiate from within, you must get to know your body on its own terms.

How? Learn its language. The body does not speak English. It speaks food, rest, movement, and touch. Those are its native tongues, and yours to master too, for the purpose of creating a dialogue and thereby a relationship with your body.

Because your body is unique, it will have experiences it enjoys and responds well to. There's no point in fretting about what your body isn't, or doesn't do. Better to spend your time getting to know the one body you have, honestly and without any delusions or fantasies. Revere the fact that there will never be another one like yours! Be in awe of the probability that you came to inhabit it—a slight probability, if you really consider the odds of reproduction. It's really quite amazing.

> *The body does not speak English.*

The following is a guide to the body's native languages.

Body Language #1: Get Right with Food!

Food is sustenance, and it's also one of the great pleasures of modern life. Never in the history of the human species have we had so much delicious food so readily available to us! We should be able to use food both as medicine *and* delight.

There are many modern ideas about how to eat, and there's always a new fad. Who knows: one might work for you! Some simple considerations, however, can make a big difference. Reflect on these three factors.

- How much you eat

- When you eat

- What you eat

How Much You Eat

For the fortunate majority in economically prosperous nations, food is so abundant that we've become unable to identify a "portion." Sometimes packaging is deceptive. You buy a "small" bag of chips, only to discover that it contains two portions. No fair!

We often use food for purposes besides sustenance and pleasure. Many of us use it to manage our emotions. Anxious? Eat. Lonely? Eat! Angry? Eat! Feeling unloved? *Eat!*

These behaviors warp our perception of fullness because often no amount of food can fill the emotional emptiness within. As an emotional overeater, I ate my emotions. Jenny Craig recalibrated my relationship with portion sizes, and I was shocked to discover it's about one-third of what we generally consume.

While sorting out my relationship with food, I swapped out junk for quality. It was a commitment I made to myself to "eat well." But improved food quality didn't address my portion misperceptions, and I found myself eating entire pots of brown rice and whole bunches of celery. Overeating is still overeating, even if the food of choice is "healthy." Alas.

When it comes to how much to eat, some of us restrict, afraid we'll eat too much. For most of us, if we restrict too much it means that we are headed straight for an overeating meltdown. Restriction is a pathway to binging. Some make restriction a way of life, becoming lifelong "career anorexics."

Overeating is still overeating, even if the food of choice is "healthy."

While I don't advocate diets per se, because it's difficult-to-impossible to disentangle prescriptive eating from diet culture, it's true that some people need to be taught how to eat by being *told* precisely what, how much, and when to eat. Whether we eat too much or eat too little, our relationship to food can get so messed up we're no longer able to decipher our body's hunger and satiety signals. The simple question *how much to eat* becomes an uncertain quagmire. We use food as a replacement for love, connection, feeling, acceptance, and the nutrition that we are gravely lacking in other areas of our lives. In this emotional or spiritual state, how much to eat becomes a labyrinth impossible to navigate.

Sometimes having a prescription for what to eat helps us get on the right track while simultaneously freeing up the mental bandwidth we've used thinking about food, so we can instead connect to the emotions bound up in our relationship with food and think about the nutritional value of our lives on the whole. If you think you need a prescriptive diet, I recommend you find someone clinically trained in both nutrition *and* some kind of psychology, with an eating disorder specialty, so they can help you with both aspects simultaneously.[41]

Restriction is a pathway to binging.

Finally, notice whether the quantity that you eat—or don't eat—is somehow a stand-in for the *size* of life that you desire—or fear. We women are told to tame our appetites, not just for food, but also for success, sex, money, love, and accolades, to name a few. Sometimes the food becomes a proxy for wanting more but not feeling like we can have it. Is your appetite for food a surrogate for your appetite for life? What if you "fed" yourself the experiences you honestly long for, instead of indulging in or denying yourself food? Sometimes this feels impossible. Don't give up! What is the smallest step you can take to address your life longings head on?

When You Eat

Increasingly, scientific evidence supports the notion that our internal organs function best a certain times of the day, aligned with circadian rhythms. Organs are not machines—they need to rest too!

Studies show that, in every organ, thousands of genes switch on and off at roughly the same times every day. A growing body of research demonstrates that chronically disrupting our circadian rhythms—by eating late meals or nibbling on midnight snacks, for example—could lead to metabolic trouble.[42] And most of the evidence in human studies suggests that consuming the bulk of your food earlier in the day is better for your health. Numerous studies demonstrate that blood sugar control is best in the morning and worst in the evening. We burn more calories and digest food more efficiently in the morning as well.[43]

Given this information about circadian rhythms, here are sensible guidelines to the basic question "When should I eat?"

1.   Make lunch your biggest meal.

2.   Eat regular meals: breakfast, lunch, dinner, perhaps with a snack in there somewhere that helps your blood sugar levels stay steady, if need be.

That's basically it. Simple, right?

Well, it's not so simple when you think about the question differently.

When do you eat?

- When I'm lonely

- When I'm sad

- When I'm angry

- When I'm bored

- When I'm horny

- When I'm tired

- When I wake up in the middle of the night besieged by all of my worst fears

- I eat a lot at parties in order to avoid talking to people, except about my deep abiding love of cheese

- When I'm watching TV

- In the car, driving

- I eat a lot, really fast, by myself, standing over the sink

- When I think no one is looking

- At 4 a.m.

- When I'm alone

- I definitely never eat on dates—well, maybe only salads

- I try to never eat

These are all emotional and existential challenges you'll need to address head on, courageously, each on its own terms. Using food to soothe or calm or avoid our emotions is like trying to use a hammer to cut down a tree. It's the wrong tool for the job, and it just makes things worse!

It's not your fault! We have very good reasons for all of our messed-up food issues. As women, we're so often denied our emotions. We've been taught for centuries that our emotions make us the "weaker sex." In order to not be "weak," we learn to manage our feelings in creative ways, like with food.

Do this instead. When you feel like eating (or starving yourself) for any of these misplaced reasons, try to discover what would *actually* help. Review the Formula for Change. To catch yourself, stop and sit down. Take ten deep breaths. Congratulate yourself for catching the behavior and reward yourself lavishly. Then ask yourself: what is the first step that I could take to help myself in a healthy direction?

Here are some tools you can use to talk to your emotions in their own language.

1. Move your body: run, dance, swim, spin, jump rope, box, wrestle, do yoga! Anything that helps touch your emotional body. Explore matching the movement with the emotion you might need released. Anger and aggression have a different channel than sadness or loneliness.

2. Listen to music; sing out loud. Cry! Yell!

3. Make art—any kind will do. Draw, cook (yes, sometimes this is how people shift their relationship with food), knit, throw pots. You choose!

4. Meditate.

5. Clean your house—you might be surprised what the activity of moving and cleaning will do for you.

6. Pull some weeds from the garden, rake leaves, mow the lawn, chop wood. Manual labor can be quite cathartic!

7. Call a friend who is sure to understand and help. Don't make the mistake of calling the wrong friend. Not everyone is the right person to help you with your emotions.

8. Watch funny movies—laughing will help move the energy!

9. Watch inspirational videos. I have a queue of them on Facebook for when I need a good cry. Crying helps release emotions and shifts your body chemistry.

10. Masturbate. Yup, I said it! An orgasm can change your mood fast!

11. Sleep. Sometimes a good long night of sleep can help you shift your perspective.

12. Nap. Even a short shot of sleep can change everything!

One of my students recently recounted to me how she used her deep breathing to help herself out of a bout of anxiety. I had just told her about being blindsided by a breakup. She asked if I used my deep breathing to help myself feel better. I said, no, actually, I really *allowed* myself to have the feelings. This is another way to break the habit of using food to manage our emotions. What if we were to feel them—and be okay feeling them?

Sometimes you need to handle your emotions *fast*—say, you're headed into a business meeting and just got some bad news on the phone. Can you compartmentalize for a moment, do your job, and *then* really allow yourself to feel?

Sometimes we need to find ways to allow ourselves to feel our emotions. Give yourself the day off to grieve a loss. Give yourself the day off to celebrate a triumph! The important point is that we learn to handle our emotions with tools that speak directly to them and to our bodies, which do the job of feeling our emotions.

All this takes work, and I think that once we have a disordered relationship with food and our emotions, chances are we'll experience it to some degree for the rest of our lives. Chances are high it'll show up again in big, stressful, positive or negative periods of life—like starting a new education, relationship, job, or experiencing a breakup, job loss, illness, or death. If you begin to see the signs and handle them like this—*Oh, it's been ages since I ate an entire sixteen-ounce bag of M&Ms in a sitting. Huh—I wonder what I'm upset about that I'm not giving myself space to really feel?*—then you're learning to handle yourself skillfully and course-correct more quickly, allowing space and attention for your own emotions.

Here are some signs that you might be getting over your emotional eating habits, learning to feel emotions, and handling them on their own terms.

- Eating (or restricting!) is no longer the answer to any unidentifiable or uncomfortable sensation in the physical or emotional body. Tired—sleep. Sad—cry. Happy—laugh. Upset—talk to a friend. Horny—get it on! Overly restless—move the body. Low back hurts—explore how to relieve its suffering.

- Eating food (or restricting!) for the wrong reasons feels unsatisfying or even disappointing.

- When you wake up in the middle of the night, you acknowledge your feelings instead of further denying them, or numbing them with food. How? You make a note to resolve the problem the next day. Craft the message to whomever you're upset with, but don't send it. Or you get up and *do* the task you're concerned about.

- At parties, instead of hanging out by the chips, cheese, or drinks, you can face social anxiety head on and do something about it.

Remember that your emotions are the source of your greatest wisdom. When you feel them—instead of eating them!—you are doing the brave work of being embodied. What beautiful contributions—art, relationships, businesses—can you produce as the result of your emotions? Who can you *be* if you honor the truth of your emotions? These are the prizes that await you when you embody your self. They are worth it.

What You Eat

Finding out what your body really thrives on—not what you *think* it likes to eat, or what someone told you is healthy—is an ongoing, lifelong process. Because, well, as you change, you change. It also is part of an embodied path. It's empowering to take ownership and responsibility for your body! Discovering what your body truly likes to eat will be impossible if you haven't first developed a relationship *with* it. You've got to start somewhere!

Begin by paying attention to how your body reacts to what you eat. Sometimes we *think* a food is a good idea, but when we actually eat it the results aren't wonderful. Pay attention to how you feel while eating, immediately after eating, and within two hours of eating. Here are some signs your body might not like what you've consumed:

- Flushing

- Fatigue

- Headaches

- Stomach pain

- Poor concentration

- Shakiness

- Feeling light-headed or spacy

Become a detective. When you eat, what are the true and real results? How is your energy? How are your bowels? Yes, your poop. It will tell you a lot!

It should be common knowledge by now that manufactured and processed foods are suboptimal for your body. Yes, they are certainly convenient and designed to satisfy humans' basic cravings for the sweet, fat, and salty (and crunchy or creamy)—but they are rarely nutritious and are often filled with chemicals and additives that aren't "food" and may even be toxic. Eat less, or none at all. Instead, cook for yourself more! What are your favorite dishes? Could you teach yourself to make them?

A simple guideline that will quickly improve your health is to *eat less sugar.* It's in just about everything that comes prepared or in a box and even shows up in places it's certainly not needed. Why, you might ask? Because it makes the food we eat addictive. Investigative journalists have recently revealed that food manufacturers purposefully design food to circumvent all the body's natural inclinations to stop when full.[44] The sugar industry lied, making us believe eating fat made us fat.[45] Nothing could be farther from the truth.[46]

So, once you've done these two things:

- Eat fewer processed and commercially prepared foods.

- Eat less sugar.

You'll be doing your body good.

Here are a few more tips, as you make any dietary adjustments:

- Go slow. Don't change too many things at once. Tackle *just one* thing at a time and do your best to stick with it.

- Swap out lower-quality foods for higher-quality foods. If you have a hankering for a particular treat—pizza, chocolate, cookies—become a connoisseur and eat only the very best.

- Make sure your choices are sustainable. Ask yourself, *could I eat this way for the next five years and enjoy it?*

- Adopt the 85/15 rule. Eat the best you can 85 percent of the time. The other 15 percent, enjoy and indulge in those high-quality treats! Life is short. Food is one of the great pleasures of modern living!

Finally, notice if the foods you eat are substitutes for other pleasures of living that you feel are lacking in your life. Find out if you can satisfy those deficiencies on their own terms. Joy comes in many forms. Food is just one of them.

Food is probably the biggest entrapment in our body confidence journey, because we *must* eat to live (whereas we don't *have* to drink alcohol or smoke), and we so closely associate what and how much we eat with diets to be thin and beautiful and therefore deserving of love, success, and all the good things in life. Don't get bogged down here! Food is just one way to take care of your body on your way to embodying your own personal truth. Keep your eyes on the prize! Getting to know your body, on its own terms, is the path to embodiment.

> *Food is just one way to take care of your body on your way to embodying your own personal truth.*

Body Language #2: Assess Your Rest!

Your body needs its rest! Getting to know your body requires discovering how much sleep you *really* need for all parts of you to fully be rested, repaired, and at their best. This isn't a thought exercise. It's not about how much you *think* you need, but how much your body *actually* needs.

So what's right for you? How would you know?

To determine whether you might be sleep-deprived, ask yourself these questions:

- Do I need an alarm clock to wake up at the right time?

- Do I have trouble getting out of bed every morning?

- Do I easily get sleepy when driving?

- Do I have trouble remembering things or concentrating?

- Do I fall asleep as soon as I get into bed?

If you answer yes to any of these questions, chances are you're not getting enough sleep. But beyond these simple diagnostics, sleep problems are much deeper embodiment problems.

Sleep Challenges and Solutions

According to the CDC, one in three Americans is sleep-deprived.[47] It happens in so many ways—staying up too late, waking up in the middle of the night and not being able to get back to sleep, or having to wake up too early.

We've got to figure this out! Sleep is *the most vital* nutrient for your body! It increases our capacity to heal, through ensuring efficient functioning of our white blood cells, which helps prevent sickness. While we sleep our memories consolidate, improving our cognitive capacities for information retention and recall.

People report that sleep is what provides the juice to be their best selves. (And the next best thing often is yoga. Seriously!)

Sleep deprivation causes our whole being to feel stressed (it *is* a torture method, after all!), which can bring on severe mental and physical problems such as depression, cardiovascular disorders, and high blood pressure. When we're sleep-deprived, we're more susceptible to misidentifying all manner of sensations. For instance, I used to mistake that "tired because I didn't get enough sleep" feeling for a generally tired feeling and would try to use food to solve the problem. Do you ever try solving your sleep problems with food or a caffeinated beverage? It just doesn't work! Sleep deprivation causes the body to crave foods with higher calorie and carbohydrate content to make up for lack of energy. No wonder potato chips seem like a great idea when you're tired! Lack of sleep also decreases metabolism at a rate that mimics the metabolic rates of aging.[48] Beauty sleep isn't just a myth!

Also, it's when we're asleep that the body repairs muscles and other tissues and improves its functioning. Sleep is essential for your body to be and do its best.

When we don't get enough sleep, we lose the capacity to be the best version of ourselves—patient, kind, generous, tolerant. It affects our relationships at home, at work, and out and about. We're more prone to anger and frustration, we struggle to pay attention, and eventually we experience overall mental exhaustion—just to mention a few of the potential horrible consequences. Daytime drowsiness decreases our alertness and can be downright dangerous. We are surely putting ourselves at risk—and we might also be endangering others!

When I don't get enough sleep, I feel like I'm pretending at everything. I'm pretending to be present. I'm pretending to teach. I'm pretending to listen. I'm pretending to care. But I'm *actually not really there.* I'm disembodied. I'm actually floating outside of my body, which is just struggling to get through the day without anyone noticing that I'm not really there. I bet you know what I'm talking about. Doing this for too long takes its toll.

Who are you able to be when you get enough sleep? When you are able to be that best version of yourself, what are you able to do?

When I am *patient,* I'm able to *be a better parent.*

When I am *kind,* I'm able to *make the people around me feel good and get better results.*

Do you see what I mean?

In your journal, complete a few for yourself. Title this page "Who Sleep Allows Me To Be."

When I'm _____, I'm able to _____.

When I'm _____, I'm able to _____.

Some of my clients have trouble getting to bed early enough to get enough sleep. Often, evening is the only time that we really have to ourselves. If you notice that you are shortchanging sleep to have some private time, or alone time, or unstructured time, can you build that into other areas of your life so you can prioritize sleep? Sometimes I realize that I've not gotten enough zoning out time, but I *know* that the sleep is more important, and I've just got to sleep!

For some people it's not so much about private time or alone time, as it is about time management. What time do you really need to be in bed to fall asleep in time to get the sleep you need? Calculate how much time prior to that you need to prepare for bed. I know that if I want to be in bed and maybe even asleep by 10:30, I need to start winding things down at 10. It might take you longer!

What do you need to help you fall sleep and stay asleep? Long ago I taught myself to sleep at night as a depression-management tool. I usually nod off instantly. But I also have some tricks for sleep hygiene when I run into trouble.

- Read fiction before bed. Story-telling is an age-old technique for putting people to sleep! Nothing too interesting! A bad book might be best, actually.

- Blackout shades or an eye mask. Make it really dark! Modernity is bright, and that tells us to be awake. Darkness tells our bodies to *go to sleep.* Shut down all the screens and devices, so nothing is illuminated.

- Aromatherapy. Diffuse oils, or use a tissue scented with a soothing sleep blend, placed on or under your pillow (see the Resources Guide).

- White noise. There are a number of apps for cueing up white noise on your phone. But in general, it's a good idea to keep your sleeping space clear of stimulation, like computers, phones, and yes, even televisions!

- Relaxation music. I have a favorite album I've been listening to for *years,* Stargarden's album *Ambient Excursions.*

- Nature sounds. Waves. Rain. Wind. Crickets. Usually these come in the white noise app.

- People talking. Sometimes, when I try all these tricks, and nothing works, I'll turn on a podcast. A long, one, talking about history or economics. Or, an audio book can work too. Make sure it's nothing you actually *really* care about enough to pay attention to!

If you wake up in the middle of the night, you might check your caffeine consumption. Too much coffee or tea can disturb your sleep. If anxious thoughts awaken you, sit up, get out of bed, get a journal, and start writing down everything rattling around in your head. Empty it out so that it's not poking you when your defenses are down. If you're certain you're going to forget something, make lists.

Sometimes unprocessed emotions disturb us in the middle of the night. Usually, my anger wakes me up. I've penned excellent emails and texts in at 3 a.m. (but never sent them)! If you do this, save as a draft; check your writing again during daylight hours to make sure it conveys your sincerest, most noble self, and then decide whether to send. If unprocessed emotions chronically plague you and keep you awake, consider getting a therapist, or if you already have one, diving in deeper in your sessions.

Additionally, if you're bothered by waking in the middle of the night for an extended period of time—like months—consider that something existential might be plaguing you. Like: *What are you doing with this one precious life!?* This could be a good question to journal on. Also, the witching hour isn't called that for no reason. Between the hours of 2 and 4 a.m. and peaking at 3 a.m., this is a time when spirits, ancestors, and sacred and eternal ones of all varieties might be trying to communicate with you. Ask if there is something you need to know, something that they are trying to tell you.

If you're struggling with nighttime rest, consider having some in the middle of the day. A short nap, lying down and putting your legs up against the wall, or even a twenty-minute meditation can restore some energy.

Take sleep seriously! It's a realm at the intersection of our bodies and our spirits. Enough, and we can be embodied spirits. Not enough and we become disembodied husks. Finally, if you really can't get a handle on this, consider seeing a medical sleep specialist, or hiring a yoga therapist to assist you. Sleep is beyond critical to your health.

What's enough sleep for you? What steps can you take to improve your sleep hygiene tonight? If my recommendations don't help, consider seeing a sleep specialist. It's *that* important. Take care of your body by giving it the rest it needs, so that you can be the best version of yourself and live your best life.

Body Language #3: Movement and Touch

Many Americans dutifully go to the gym. But, if you honestly consider it, do you really enjoy going to the gym? Does your body shiver with pleasure while running on the treadmill? Does your mind feel engaged by the activities that you choose at the gym?

Chances are you go to the gym out of a sense of moral obligation. (For those of you who honestly don't—brava!)

I was a gym rat for a long time. I worked out in some capacity, seven days a week, for many years. But I did so for the entirely wrong reasons. I did so out of a wish to tame, control, and forestall what I perceived to be the increasing unruliness of my body. I was disgusted by it, and the gym was my control measure. This approach is incorrect.

Consider the best approach to training an animal. Shaming it into compliance, or terrorizing it into obedience is never a long-lasting approach. You may get immediate results, but the core of the method is rotten. Not only is it cruel and destructive, but it will make the animal crazy.

It's the same with training your body. If you shame it, abuse it, or self-mutilate with lacerating thoughts, the body will rebel, and the person within warps and starts to go mad. The body rebels through defense mechanisms like injury, illness, rapid deterioration, and becoming too thin or too heavy. The spirit within sickens too.

I'm very familiar with all of the crazy "exercise" we do in the name of so-called health. This I can tell you from first-hand experience: although working out is great, doing things you hate out of obligation while thinking how ugly and disgusting the body is—that's self-abuse.

When I finally came to terms with my seven-days-a-week exercise habit for what it truly was—a form of self-mutilation—I stopped. And I sat on my ass. And I rested. Because goodness knows, I was tired from that two-hours-every-day routine, combined with a starvation regimen! And my mind was exhausted from managing all those horrible things I would say to myself repeatedly while exercising.

While I rested, interestingly enough, I lost weight. I'm not saying that this is a laudable outcome; I'm pointing out that the body mostly doesn't work the way that we've been told it does. Meaning: exercise doesn't always lead to weight loss. Surprise!

Science writer Gary Taubes points out the delusional, magical thinking we commonly engage in: that working out will help us lose weight. Actually, there's little supporting evidence for the belief that burning up calories has any effect on how fat we are.[49] Working out makes us hungry and often leads us to eat more than we might have otherwise. Says Taubes, "Increase the energy that you expend and the evidence is very good that you will increase the calories that you consume to compensate."[50]

Exercise doesn't always lead to weight loss.

So, honestly, if you abandoned the idea that working out makes you lose weight, would you still do it?

I'm not advocating that we become (more) sedentary. I'm pointing out how often our *reasons* for moving our bodies are founded on wrong perceptions and misplaced motivations. Movement—one of the body's primary pleasures—has been reframed for women as something compulsory we need to do to stay thin and therefore be good and valuable. Something innocent, wonderful, and beautiful was taken away and sold back to us as a moral obligation.

Doing anything out of fear, hate, or the idea that you will avoid some horrible fate as a result—this is incorrect thinking. It is a form of oppression.

Doing the things that you do out of love, trust, and enjoyment—this is correct thinking. It is also a form of freedom.

After a number of years of not formally exercising at all, I found yoga. This began what is to date an almost twenty-year exploration of a physical activity.

I do it not because I'm required to. I do it not because I think that I will be thin or look younger as a result. I do it out of the sheer pleasure that the activity gives my body, and the stimulation that it provides my mind. I'm not saying that the mind-set of using yoga for "exercise" or weight loss didn't ever creep in—it has, and it still does. The idea that movement should be for material beautification purposes is so prevalent and we are so deeply steeped in it, and have been for so long, it will *always* be there to seduce us.

Our intent for selecting what we do is of utmost importance, and we are free to choose. You can't tell why a person is lifting weights just from looking at them. For instance, after nearly twenty years of "not working out" I realized that the needs of my body have shifted dramatically and changed. It *needs* what the gym has to offer. Lifting things, pushing and pulling heavy weights is what it was calling for. Getting back in the pool and swimming for an hour, uninterrupted. This is what it's been crying out for. I felt a little bit like an alcoholic going to a bar—could I do it without going back to my habit of too much too often while hating myself? After twenty years, a lot of therapy and as much yoga, the answer was *yes*. My intent has changed dramatically. I use the gym for me, and to fulfill my body's true longings and desires, not to feed an addiction. The gym—just like a scale, or a mirror, or a doughnut, or a stalk of celery—is empty of meaning. We are the ones who imbue anything with meaning. The object or activity is inert.

The fun, empowerment, and responsibility of living embodied lies in constantly listening to the body and responding to its communications. This is the art of relationship. Listen; respond. This is how we build trust, and also that thing that we all say we want and desire in life: unconditional love. This is the way you gift it to yourself. By getting to know your body, truly and honestly, on its own terms.

I love yoga—it's taught me so much—but as a form of movement, it may not be your jam. Find a physical practice that you truly enjoy. Find two or three. You can choose how you think and feel about your body and the activities that influence your thinking. Study your motives and how the movement feels to your body. Choose wisely!

What movement practices do you particularly enjoy? List five of them in your journal. Title your page "Movement My Body Enjoys." Look, I'll start.

- Horseback riding, on trails. I *love* being outside! With horses!

- Swimming. I *love* the feeling of the water on my skin! *Yum.*

- I love hitting and kicking things. Most recently I'm learning Krav Maga.

Your turn! Keep going, in your journal.

Everyday Touch

One of the things many people love about yoga is being touched. Some yoga teachers touch more than others. Some never do. If you consent, and if the touch is kind, generous, and clean (meaning free of any expectation or sexual charge), it can be tremendously healing for the body and the being within.

Touch is a vital nutrient for your body and a fundamental language. Too many of our bodies are starving for this nourishment and form of communication. My teacher Ana Forrest trains us to touch our students "as if we are touching the Beloved." What she means by this is, whenever I as a yoga teacher have an opportunity to touch a person, I am touching the divine, and I should treat touching with that degree of reverence.

The body knows the meaning and the intent behind touch. I've found that my students often need to be reeducated that they can trust touch. I'll put my hands on them and they will tense up, anticipate, resist, or even fight. The moment I say, "Listen to my hands, they're allies; they're talking to you" they relax and use a different part of their intelligence to comprehend what I'm communicating. The shift is almost always immediate as they go into listening, receiving, and cocreating from the body's intelligence.

Dr. Betty Martin has developed an in-depth body of knowledge, articulating the fundamental concepts of learning about touch: giving, taking, receiving, and allowing. The other four metrics are giving, doing, receiving, and done-to. Combined, these create her Wheel of Consent. To really learn about touch, I recommend Dr. Martin's courses and materials (see the Resource Guide).

Touch is vitally important! We are hardwired to thrive, mentally, emotionally, and physically on loving touch. So where are we to acquire this essential nutrient for our bodies?

Here are some ideas. Some prioritize receiving, some are a mixture of giving and receiving.

- Restorative yoga, yin yoga, Forrest Yoga are all styles that prioritize kind, generous, clean touch.

- Massage, reiki, craniosacral therapy—there are so many kinds of body workers in the world, you could spend a lifetime exploring what modalities you enjoy for the sheer pleasure of receiving touch.

- Dance! I've found that so much of what people enjoy about dance is the opportunity to engage physically in a safe space with other people. Partner dances have rules, so you know what to do and what not to do. This can be fun and satisfying for the body and for your spirit.

- Try AcroYoga or other kinds of partner yoga. These are spaces where people find out about the body together, explore clear and safe communication, and consciously investigate the ways that people create healthy relationships. These kinds of yoga also emphasize both giving *and* receiving touch.

- Fight! Our bodies have impulses to do many things, and fighting may be among them. This can also be a safe and structured way to touch and engage with other people and their bodies while at the same time empowering your body to know that you can defend it and be safe within it. There are so many forms of fighting that can be fun and exhilarating. Boxing, MMA, jujitsu, Krav Maga, fencing. Some of them involve sparring, others don't. You can find out!

- Get a blowout, a wash'n'dry, or a manicure!

- Hire a cuddlist. Yes—you can get someone to come over and do whatever you want, as long as it is nonsexual![51]

- Solo self-touch is also helpful. Showers, washing your hair, massaging oil or lotion into your skin, dry brushing your skin, self-reiki, and masturbation all fall into this category. There's a lot to explore on your own, if involving another person doesn't feel good.

Does something on this list look doable to you? Which one? Or, is there something you would prefer that's *not* on the list?

Start to catalog what your body likes in your journal. Title your page, "Touch My Body Likes and Needs."

Sexual Touch

Often through experience we've been taught that touch comes in two categories— violent or sexualized. Sometimes those categories overlap. Too often, men may find that they're simply never touched at all except in a sexual capacity. Consider how freely women can touch one another. We hug, snuggle, and pet one another. We visit the hairdresser and the manicurist. Men can't freely do the same without enduring negative cultural connotations.

Inevitably, in my coaching program when we get to the module covering movement and touch, the subject of intimate relations arises. This is a high-tension, fraught conversation for women who feel their bodies are undesirable. The fear of judgment, rejection, and disappointment can be overwhelming, and an unwillingness to take off your clothes and be seen naked could understandably stall the advancement of any intimate relationship. Here, in one of the most vulnerable acts we can undertake as women (sex!) is the dazzlingly complex intersection of

- Our right to be our authentic selves, no matter the shape or size of our bodies

- The longing for love and intimate partnership

- Our body's need to be touched

What an overwhelming confluence of issues! What can you do?

Unflinchingly, be who you are right now, explore who you are inside and out, define and develop who you are, and put that out in the world unapologetically. When you're authentically yourself, you attract people who see you for who you are; then, when you take off your clothes, they are attracted to *you* as a person. Above all, don't disguise your body!

I recall watching a video made by some fat activists I enjoy following who said basically: "*Girl!* He *knows* you're fat! He *knows* what he signed up for! So—take off your clothes already!!!" One lover was relieved that I didn't "fall apart" when I took off my clothes. Meaning— slimming underwear is false advertising. These garments make everyone *more* anxious about getting naked! Consider going without body-shaping undergarments.

Virgie Tovar noticed, in her coaching programs for women who want to break up with diet culture, that it's at the moment when the question of intimacy arises that many women lose their resolve and go back to dieting. The most important factor for their continued progress was the ability to envision a future with a partner who was either fat-positive or queer.[52]

Regardless of your gender identity or sexual orientation, finding a body-positive partner is key! From all that I know on the heterosexual front, I believe that men love women's bodies with far more interest and wide-ranging curiosity than we're taught to believe. If you're a woman seeking a male partner, how can you find one who is interested in women of all shapes and sizes?

1. *Be* the woman of whatever shape and size you are. When you are that person, you will attract people who are interested in the truth of who and what you are. When you attract people who like the real version of you, that allows you to be yourself in front of them at all times.

2. Study the way that he reacts to other women, talks about women's bodies, talks about women's potential and place in the world.

3. Find out whether he celebrates women's happiness and wants to support women's growth as human beings. You can accomplish this by asking questions about his understanding and feelings about his mother, sisters, aunts, female friends, and female coworkers. Better yet, if he already has children, explore his hopes for his sons or daughters. What kind of a life does he desire for them?

4. Pay attention to a man's first reaction to your body. Go for the guy who likes you just the way you are.

When a man loves women and women's bodies (and you love a man and men's bodies!), chances are the movement and touch aspect of your relationship (sex!) will be more satisfying.

Whatever way feels safe, inviting, and comfortable to you, continue to educate yourself about touch so that you can be fully embodied and therefore be the best rendition of *you*. Touch is a critical aspect of your body's health and therefore of *your* health. For some people, touch *is* the way to embodiment. It might be for you too.

Many of these movement and touch activities assume that you are well and able-bodied. We'll all be sick at some point in time, some of us live with physical challenges that begin early in our lives, and our ability to move and touch may be greatly diminished in the future. What's important is that we explore these vital areas of life in whatever way we are able to. I live with a chronic illness. Sometimes the best I can do is

The body is the way in, to everything.

walk to the kitchen or take a bath. It might be nice to have someone around to rub my feet or my back too. If we're able to notice these longings, it's the first step to fulfilling them. Without our embodied relationship we might not even be able to hear the call; then the body goes on starving for the nutrition it really needs. Sometimes a foot rub or back rub is medicine for the spirit and the soul, not just the body.

Your body is unique. The beauty you generate and emanate is your distinction, created from your own interaction *with* your body, its preferences, and your life circumstances. Treat your body with the reverence it deserves, and dive into the mystery of what makes it thrive. When you do, you'll see that everything about you starts to change, and as you come to know yourself completely and thoroughly, you will begin to understand what makes you distinct and live in that reality. The genuineness of engaging in your own mystery will be utterly enchanting, and should pull your attention away from fantasies of wishing to have the body of the 4 percent.

Your body is beyond statistics! There will never, ever be another being like you, and that is worth being awed about. Treat your body as such.

Self-Care Is Sacred

In yoga we have a practice called *sadhana*. Sadhana means daily spiritual practice. It is the foundation of all spiritual endeavors; your personal, individual spiritual effort. It's the main tool you use to work on yourself to achieve the purpose of life. I believe that in addition to using our sankalpah, which manages and focuses the energy of our minds and our intentions, we also need a sadhana that supports our belief that the body is the center of our spiritual endeavors and the path, the way, and the light to finding our purpose for life. Therefore, it is important to do something daily that centers the pleasure and acceptance of the body. I assign you this spiritual homework, once assigned to me by Ana Forrest: do one thing a day that delights your spirit. Get to know *you* with this question in mind: what makes you distinct? What do you need to provide for yourself, today, to support the growth of your one, singular, utterly unique body? What is it about you that is so utterly unreplicable that you have no other choice but to stand in awe of the rarity of your being? Be astonished!

We're nearing the end of our journey together, dear reader. I hope, with all of my heart, that you've been altered, in the way that makes people who have long known you do a double take, wondering *what's changed?* Because the more you transform your insides—your thoughts and beliefs about yourself and the world around you—the more it shows up on your outside in a shimmering, ineffable radiance we call *beauty.*

In the final lesson, we'll look at how to know the rest of your self through the etheric *koshas,* and we'll start to use your body to mine for answers to the most important questions of your life. This work thrills me, and the *way* of doing it—employing the body as the instrument of discovery—feels so honest and true I almost can't contain my excitement for you! So turn the page, and let's begin to unearth your answers. They will transform you, for the better, forever.

You Are More Than Your Body

Recently I had a staph infection. I skinned my knee on my yoga mat and didn't bother to cover the wound. It healed up, but later little bumps filled with clear fluid appeared on my knee. Still later, an abscess developed. I self-treated and prevailed, but another appeared. Finally, after having a friend look at it, I went to the doctor. She was stern with me. She drew on my leg, marking a perimeter around the oozing wound.

"If the swelling goes outside these lines tonight, you must go to the emergency room. If there are any red steaks on your leg, you must go to the emergency room. *Whenever* the dermatologist has time for you tomorrow, you *must* go. Okay?" I nodded in glum agreement.

Looking dejectedly at the knee, I realized the bacteria was liquefying it. I began considering life without a leg. I would survive. Probably. The leg might not. But even without a leg, I would still be me. Right?

Of course, the experience would change me forever—the "me" we call the body, and the rest of "me" that would endure the experience alongside the body. But the contours of my life, those determined by my body, would be indelibly altered. Would I still be able to get around New York City to teach? Would my students still view me as fit enough to do so? It's tricky to escape definitions that describe "me" as my material form. But no matter what happened, I would still be myself.

BODY IMAGE IS A MENTAL CONSTRUCT

One of the great, enduring questions posed to aspiring contemplatives and meditators is: *What are you?*

If the question functions as intended, it should bring an abrupt halt to your regular, habituated thinking. Suddenly, we are groundless, left grasping thin air. *Hmmmmm. How to answer?* Well now, tell me: what are you? Let's make a list right now, in your journal. Ten things you are. *Go!* Write at the top of your page: *Ten Things I Am.* Then list away!

So much of our society is bent on convincing us we're our wardrobe, our cool haircut, our job, our car, or the contents of our bank account. In modern times, this time-honored question—what are you?—means more. It also asks *what value do you have?*

We know, we know! We've got it by now! Women are valuable for being pretty, snagging a man, and having babies. Men are valuable for being strong and productive and attaining status. Failing one or the other, you're worthless. A loser.

This line of reasoning lies at the core of so much modern suffering. When society values materialism and commodities, it logically follows that society will also place its highest value on a person's material aspect—the body. But are you your body?

Immediate logic says, *well of course I'm my body, because if I die (meaning if my body dies), then I am no more.* It's impossible to prove human consciousness exists apart from a living body.

But we understand, more instinctually than we're aware of, that we're not *just* our bodies. When a person dies, we say, *their body* lies in the coffin. (Or more commonly these days, in the urn.) Where, then, has the person who once resided within that body gone? Our sense of self is innately quite malleable.

When a woman is pregnant, suddenly her concept of "body" extends to include another being. This sense endures long after the physical bodies of the mother and child have separated. Parents will defend their children with their lives, because their children's lives are literally an extension of their own. Children are our legacy. Through procreation we become "immortal." Some people describe their children—even those they did not create biologically!—as "having my heart walking around outside of me." As a parent, what you label "you" is no longer contained within the boundaries of your own skin. How can that be?

This curiosity also works inversely. Imagine you're diabetic; your toes lose circulation, becoming gangrenous, and must be amputated. If they're not severed, they'll die, and the decaying flesh will poison the rest of the body and threaten its survival. Under these circumstances, we must shrink our idea of "self" to exclude those toes. We feel the loss, to be sure, but nonetheless will sacrifice the body to save the self. Living in a diminished container seems a small concession.

Similarly, when you want to lose weight, you disavow the parts of you that you dislike and want to get rid of. Some people even imagine the fat body isn't their true self; that a skinny person is trapped within, trying to escape! Think of all the times you've said I hate my...[fill in the blank]. Regardless of the shape of the body, in that moment you're acknowledging, whatever you are or may be, you're not your body.

If this is true, and the you defined by your body expands or contracts according to how you elect to think about it, and whether or not you have biological children, the body simply cannot be a reliable foundation on which to build your sense of what is you at all. Body image is the mental picture that you make of your self and project out into the world. How you think about the body establishes how you show up in the visible world. Our material form is, in many ways, a projection of our mind.

When you look inside—meaning when you direct your mind's eye inward—what do you see? Looking within my own body, I can see its structures expanding inward like a horizon, universe, and galaxies.

Body image is the mental picture that you make of yourself and project out into the world.

Let's work on deepening your body image, both inward and outward. I like to start with the bones. First read the following instructions, then try the exercise.

Imagining Inward

1. Close your eyes and draw a mental picture of the bones in your hand.

2. See them as golden and shining.

3. As you inhale, find out if you can breathe into the bones of the hand.

4. As you exhale, find out if you can breathe out from the bones of the hand.

As you gain more skill with this, you can continue to map a picture of your body from the inside. You might start by completing your skeleton in as much detail as possible and then start to add your major organs.

Now ask the question: *What am I?* and find out what answers you come up with. Continue your list in your journal, under "Ten Things I Am."

Studying the body is a mystical practice. Through these exercises I began to comprehend that a whole cosmos lies within, literally and mystically. Each cell is its own universe.

We are vast inside.

Just as quantum physics has proven our galaxy is expanding, we too are also expanding. Here's an exercise to feel into what that means.

Expanding Outward

1. Inhale and feel your torso expand.

2. Exhale and press your self outward energetically, squeezing your low abdomen back toward your spine.

3. Inhale, and as your torso expands, feel and see your self expand to the perimeter of your torso.

4. Exhale and again press your self out, energetically.

5. Inhale, and as your torso expands, again feel and see your self expand beyond the perimeter of your skin.

6. Exhale and focus on blowing and pressing your self farther, beyond the container of your physical body.

Doing this exercise, you might have difficulty taking up all the space inside of your own body. *Expanding Outward* can be a tremendously healing first step, to own and occupy all corners and pockets of your own body with your breath and awareness. It can also be confronting, because shrinking within is a way we learn to be small and therefore safe and acceptable. Challenging that notion may immediately trigger an aspect of you programmed for safety and survival. This part of you—she will come on strong. In an effort to keep you "safe," she may sabotage you, trying to make you be small again. She may program flashbacks or incredibly uncomfortable phantom somatic sensations like nausea, overwhelming sleepiness, or brain fog. Learn to recognize the difference between coming up against an internal barrier whose dismantling will benefit your growth and an actual danger to be feared and avoided. Learning this discernment prepares your to grow beyond your comfort zone and be more of who you are becoming.

Expanding Outward can also be triggering if you discover you don't own or occupy parts of your body. This raises the question *who or what is living in those spaces where you are not?* Ana Forrest calls these people and notions existing within our unoccupied regions "squatters." While you weren't paying attention and weren't home, they moved into your body. Breathing into these spaces and sending your mind into them gets you started with evicting unwanted guests and taking up residence in your own home again.

As you do this work, you may also start to have a sense of your self as bigger than your body. This can be confronting to women who've been taught "being big" is something to avoid at all costs. "Taking up space" in this way is a skill you can deploy when needed. You can expand and contract at will. When I teach, I purposefully make myself large. When stop teaching, I "turn it off." In certain situations, I'll do my best to make myself small or even invisible. You can learn to do this too; however, living small isn't the objective. Some people habitually hide by shrinking energetically within. This chronically harms the spirit. If you hide, ask yourself: from what? What danger do you fear, and what would happen to you if you stopped hiding?

Assess whether the danger is current, present, and real, or if it is a legacy of your past. Break free! Evolve, and claim your freedom.

Holding Good Boundaries

These exercises also help us explore and shore up boundaries that might be leaky. Think of it this way: if you own property and never walk the lot line, you'll be completely unaware if there's a hole in your fence. Exploring the edges of our being helps us know ourselves, stop leaking energy, and grow in the ways that feel safe and healthy to us, and it keeps out unwanted strangers. This is part of having good boundaries.

Boundaries are different from walls and armor. The latter are protective, designed to keep out people and ideas considered unwanted or dangerous. They also lock us inside. Boundaries, on the other hand, are intended to be both strong and permeable. In addition to letting in friendly visitors, they also allow *you* to move across your own perimeter at will and explore beyond. Boundaries are freeing.

Good boundaries are the foundation for the next exercise, which involves purposefully growing your sense of self beyond your own skin. If you're very sensitive or highly empathetic, this exercise depends on your already having strong and healthy boundaries. If you feel like you don't yet possess these, then keep working on *Imagining Inward* and *Expanding Outward* before you move on to the following two exercises.

Encompassing Others in Loving-Kindness

Encompassing Others is an exercise in growing your own kind feelings and goodwill into the universal truth that, despite appearances of difference and separation, we're all interconnected. After you learn to really feel yourself and your own experiences, and to grow compassion for yourself, you can begin to extend this skill to others for the good of all.

This is a traditional practice from the Shambhala Buddhist tradition, as described by Pema Chödrön, called "Loving-Kindness Meditation." The seven steps traditionally begin with expanding a feeling of goodwill for yourself, but some people find it hard to begin there. If you have difficulty extending kindness toward yourself, you could start with anything that immediately produces a feeling of goodwill within you, like a dog or a cat, or your favorite person. Don't fake a good feeling! Really bring it up, and then expand it into others. As you do this exercise, you might say the traditional words (out loud at first, then in a whisper, then silently within) "May all sentient beings enjoy happiness and the root of happiness."

1. Awaken loving-kindness for yourself. You might say, "May I enjoy happiness and the root of happiness" or put it into your own words.

2. Practice feeling happy for someone for whom you feel sincere goodwill and tenderness: "May (name) enjoy happiness or the root of happiness" (or you can choose your own words).

3. Awaken loving-kindness for a friend, again saying the friend's name and expressing the aspiration for their goodwill.

4. Practice experiencing feelings of goodwill for someone about whom you feel neutral.

5. Awaken loving-kindness for someone you find difficult or offensive.

6. Let the loving-kindness grow big enough to include all beings in the five preceding steps. This step is called "dissolving barriers." Say, "I, my beloved, my friend, the neutral person, the difficult person, all together enjoy happiness and the root of happiness."

7. Extend loving-kindness toward all beings throughout the universe. You can start close to home and widen the circle more and more.[53]

I hope that through this exercise your body image will become much more expansive, detailed, and, frankly, beautiful. Your body is so much more than your physical form. It is part of everything.

Exchanging Yourself and Others

I'm sure that you've heard the expression "Before you judge another, walk a mile in their shoes." But how does one walk in another's shoes?

In Geshe Michael Roach and Lama Christie McNally's book *The Diamond Cutter* they describe three steps to achieving supercharged empathy:

1. Educate yourself about what others need and like. This is a simple exercise in awareness that you can practice with the people around you: family, coworkers, friends. This exercise helps us start to feel others, in a healthy way.

2. Pretend to put your mind into their body, and find out what they want from the experience of being alive. The authors call this "Switching Bodies."[54]

3. The third step they call "The Rope Trick." Here, you lasso yourself and another person, imagining that the two of you are, literally, one person.

This is a very advanced practice, which ought to blow your mind and completely *explode* your idea of body image. You can actually walk in another's shoes. You might lose your mind when you do this. It's not a horrible thing to have happen. After all, the mind isn't always our friend.

If you choose to practice *Encompassing Others* and *Exchanging Yourself,* you might need some grounding afterward. Just maybe! Take some quiet time alone to rest and pull yourself back fully and completely into your own skin.

We have a very small notion of body image! I hope these exercises have exploded yours! If you were to describe yourself now, how do you see your self? *What are you?* These exercises strengthen your intellect (the fourth *kosha)* and its connection with the body, and they expand your capacity to feel inward. When you have a stronger inner center and sense of self, it's easier to withstand the pressures of the outside world.

THE BODY IS ON LOAN

The physical body belongs to the natural world, and as part of nature it's mostly out of your control.

And is it really "your" body anyway? All of the materials with which "your" body was constructed were already here on earth before you came into being. The minerals and fluids that became "you" were freely floating in the world. It's not as if your parents went to the store and bought the ingredients to build a baby. Even our ideas of ownership and natural resources are strange—how can you own a tree, or a piece of land? We own nothing. The body is a piece of nature, on loan. With this in mind, now: *What are you?*

The more I lived with these concepts, the more I understood that the disbelief I felt when looking in the mirror, the unshakable feeling of *that can't possibly be me* is *correct.* That body, that face I see gazing back—it's *not* me. And I can no longer really be certain the "self" thinking "my" thoughts is *"me"* either.

Holy smokes! What *are* we?

The error lies in thinking we're any singularity. We are vast; we are multitudes. We're D: all of the above. We strayed and got all mixed up when we began believing the puny, human thought that the divine meant *one* thing (male, perfect). Eastern thinking knows intrinsically that the creator is diversity and a greater power is everywhere and all things, and sought to represent that awareness through various and multiple beautiful and grotesque representations of spirit. The creator is male, it is female, wrathful, peaceful, and everything in between. The divine is all things. Therefore humans are all things. Most of all things, including our bodies, are out of our control. What you *can* control are your thoughts and responses to your own experiences.

> *The Divine is all things. Therefore, humans are all things.*

Here's a Thích Nhất Hạnh poem about the body as nature.

Inside is made of outside.
When we touch our own skin,
we touch the water, heat, air,
and earth that are within us.
At the same time, we know
that these elements also exist
outside our bodies.
Touching deeply,
we realize
that the sun
is also our heart.[55]

WHAT ARE YOU?

In Lesson 6 we did a deep dive into establishing a healthy relationship with your body, which is just one aspect of you but houses everything else that you are. Let's do a quick review of the koshas, the yogic model for understanding the human.

- First and most materially apparent is your food body (physical body), or *annamayakosha*. We talked about building a relationship with this part of you in lessons 4, 5, and 6.

- The second layer inward is your energy body, the *pranaymaya kosha*, which governs vital functions. We really addressed this part of you when we talked about sleep in Lesson 6 and about how you manage your energy in Lesson 3.

- Third is your mind body, *manomaya kosha*, which the yogis conceive of as finding life through the senses. We got to know our senses through the Survey of Senses in Lesson 4.

- The fourth kosha is the *vijnamayakosha*, the part of you that actively thinks, discerns, makes judgments, and possesses will. This is what we're talking about this in this lesson. In Western parlance, this aspect of you is called your "mind."

- The most esoteric part of you, which sees everything and is part of everything, the fifth veil, is the *annandamayakosha*, described as the "bliss body." We're also exploring this kosha in this chapter, especially the interplay between intellect and spirit and between these and the body.

Taking Care of You

Since you are everything, it's impossible to ever know all of you. Nonetheless, the koshas help us learn about our selves, define our selves, and take care of our selves.

How would you define yourself, knowing what you know now? In your journal, answer the following prompts. You can use the question titles as the headings for your pages.

"Defining My Self"

- What are you, materially?

- What are you, energetically?

- What are your senses?

- What are you, intellectually?

- What are you, spiritually?

Knowing now just how vast you are, can you better consider how to answer these questions?

"Taking Care of My Self"

- How can I take care of my body? (You already have a terrific head start on this from Lesson 6!)

- How can I take care of my energy and personal resources? (Look back to Lesson 6 if you need help!)

- How can I take care of my senses and my mind? (Refer to Lesson 4.)

- How can I take care of my intellect?

- How can I take care of my spirit?

- Finally, also ask this: How are they connected and overlapping? Where does taking care of one help me take care of another?

This final question is important because while the model describes the koshas as distinct, they are all housed within the body, so they are interconnected. For instance, sleep, which restores the energy body, affects the material body and the intellect too.

Taking care of your self is just the beginning of getting to know you. When you get to know you and all the ways that you experience the world and suffer, understanding, appreciation and eventually love can emerge. Learning to love your self follows this path:

Step 1: Know and understand.

Step 2: Take care (or remove suffering).

Step 3: Appreciate.

Step 4: Learn to love.

So often this last step feels like a mandate! But without education in these crucial preliminary steps, it can feel like being asked to jump off the high dive without knowing how to float! When you do the first two steps—understand and take care of your self—you'll be better prepared to answer these questions. Title your journal page: "Appreciating My Self."

- What do I appreciate about my body? What do I love about my body?

- What do I appreciate about my energy body?

- What do I appreciate about my senses and my mind?

- What do I appreciate about my intellect?

- What do I appreciate about my spirit?

The energy of appreciation encompasses the steps of understanding and taking care. When you understand yourself, you know how you suffer. Taking care of yourself, you work to remove the suffering you experience. Appreciating means to "add value." Self-appreciation means that you perceive how your experience and existence add value to the world. And finally, it prepares you to love that which you are *inside* and the person you've *become* through the process of getting to know the being you call "myself."

Our bodies aren't the problem; what and how we think about our bodies is the problem.

Knowing Your Mind

You may have discovered through reading this book that I don't believe our bodies are the real issue. Our bodies aren't the problem; what and how we think about our bodies is the problem. How we think causes tremendous suffering. Our thinking is partially the product of foibles inherent in our species and partially the result of social education, which arises circularly from our human quirks. From our thinking, our speech and actions emerge. Speech and action form our interactions with others and become the substance of our lives. When we take care of the mind, intellect, and our thinking, we're taking care of all other components of our lives as well. But as you might have also noticed, the most difficult thing to do is to change your mind.

Understanding how the human mind (the intellect) works will help you improve its health and function. Yoga is one of the earliest studies of psychology, and its purpose was to examine the ways that humans suffer and devise methods to ease it. We suffer! It's human nature to form opinions, judgments, likes, and dislikes, all of which, more often than not, contribute to our suffering. It's not your fault! This is just what we do.

The most difficult thing to do is to change your mind.

Because the mind has no form, in order to know it is real, it creates opinions.

As it presses out from within, the first material object it discovers is the body. *Your* body. And to know that it itself exists, the mind formulates a judgment about the body. Because these judgments aren't objective, they rarely are helpful, but they position us in *relationship* to other objects. Using this relativity, the mind evaluates objects and experiences as "good" or "bad." It needs to do this because any form of groundlessness means returning to a formless existence. The mind finds this prospect very frightening! It *wants* to be here, in the material world; it *wants* to be alive and experience life.

Does what I just described sound familiar to you? It's the order of the first four lessons in this book.

1. We suffer—what's the erroneous solution? *Happiness!*

2. We need to know we exist—what's the erroneous solution? *Judge and compare!*

3. We need to know we're the best—what's the erroneous solution? *Perfection!*

4. We need to know we're where we stand in the world—what's the erroneous solution? *Declare that things are good or bad!*

In each of lessons 1 through 4, you were offered an alternative mind-set to the habitual ones we've been socialized to accept. They are "replacement" mind-sets, intended to know your mind and alleviate your suffering!

When I found out that the ways I think are merely the mind's self-soothing techniques for confirming that it exists, I felt enormously liberated. Informed by this data, we don't have to take it all so seriously! You don't have to listen to the condemning, judgmental voice in your head. You can choose to ignore it, knowing what it says is mostly baseless and unhelpful. Additionally, knowing you didn't invent any of this should help absolve you of the need to blame yourself for the mess we *all* find ourselves in. None of being human is your fault! But it *is* our responsibility as evolving souls to continually educate ourselves about both society and human nature to help free ourselves from the intrinsic suffering we create and experience.

We are our minds as much as we are our bodies. This book is *mostly* designed to help you take care of your thinking. As you look back over the first four chapters, can you identify one in particular that is sticky for you? We tend to specialize in an area—for instance, I am a perfectionist (Lesson 3). I don't particularly fret about happiness, but when it comes to doing things well, being the best, I suffer a lot in that department.

What's your specialty? Make it a priority to break up the mental habits that harm you, and replace them with the ones suggested in the chapters to help you free yourself from your own suffering. Take on the lesson you most need as your primary, focused course of study.

Basic Mind-Body Health

Mind-body practices reject the machine body. Integrated practices are based on the premise that the mind and the body are connected. How could they not be? The mind lives within the body. Positively affecting the mind helps the body. Think well about yourself, and the body will react well. Positively affecting the body will help the mind. When the mind has a healthy home to live in, it tends to feel better!

A modern scientific model of the human consciousness echoes the nested rings of awareness described by the *koshas*. Science maps our quality of awareness onto brain waves—beta, alpha, theta, and delta—that describe both how quickly the energetic frequencies emitted from our brains are vibrating and the corresponding thought tendencies. Slower brainwaves = healthier mind.

To move your brainwave state from faster into slower states, practicing literally slowing down is the best way to affect your mind and open yourself up to answers. Move more slowly. Breathe more slowly. Do less. These are the ways you also retrain yourself to recognize that your value isn't exclusively in doing, but also in being.

Slowing Your Breath Duration

1. Sit still and inhale. As you do, count seconds to find out how long your inhale lasts. Then exhale, counting to find out how long your exhale lasts.

2. Now consciously make the inhale and the exhale last the same length of time. First try lengthening the shorter to match the longer. If that proves too difficult, then match the longer to the shorter length.

3. Take ten deep breaths with even inhale and even exhale.

4. Lengthen both by a count of one.

5. Continue to lengthen both by a count of one as long as you can do so easefully. When it becomes difficult or stressful, back off by a count of one and take five deep breaths at this pace.

6. Rest, breathing easily without making any effort to change the breath.

Combining breath work with yoga asana is a powerful practice and the source of virtually all my knowledge and wisdom. It came through my body! It's much more difficult to teach you yoga asana and embodiment in a book than it is to teach breathwork and meditation techniques. (See the Resource Guide for offerings.)

Interestingly enough, as the other aspects of us grow, evolve, and change, our bodies respond favorably. This should not come as a surprise. Freed up from a constant barrage of judgment, criticism, and shame, the body can begin to flourish. As a result, all of you will begin to flourish. Self-confidence is founded on confidence from *all* parts of you, including body confidence.

Again, What Are You?

It's important to take care of our thoughts, because they are the origins of how we behave. The word "behave" could be seen as the composite of two other words: "be" and "have." In other words, you have (are) what you *be*.

Thích Nhất Hạnh teaches that our only true belongings are our actions. Drawn from a Buddhist discourse, the Upajjhatthana Sutta, he articulates the Five Remembrances:

> The Buddha urged his monks to practice like this every morning. First, "I am of the nature to grow old. There is no way to escape growing old. Instead of suppressing it, invite it up, look directly at it. I am of the nature to grow old, I have to accept that." Second, "I am of the nature to have ill health. When you grow old, you will know it. There is no way to escape having ill health." [Third] "I am of the nature to die. There is no way to escape death." [Fourth] " All that is dear to me, and all that I love are of the nature to change. There is no way to escape being separated from them." Fifth, "my actions are my only true belongings. I cannot escape the consequences of my actions. My actions are the ground on which I stand."[56]

If you answered the question *What are you?* based on actions you are proud of, ones that were kind and generous to you and to others, what would be on your list?

Write on a fresh page in your journal. Title it "My Actions of Which I Am Proud." Make this list now! Go for ten items.

The genesis of your actions is thought. How you think about the world is everything. This meditation that Thích Nhất Hạnh describes is a form of "death meditation" intended to jolt us awake and to take care in our actions today. Imagine how your approach to living would change if you lived as the Buddha instructed.

It requires bravery to look at the reality of our existence. It's so heartbreaking to really see how fragile and beautiful it truly is (and we are), hurled so swiftly on a path toward death. Hopefully this truth will wake us up. We have precious little time, and we waste it in senseless ways. In light of this truth, the choice to cultivate radical acceptance and unconditional love for the one body that you have seems to me the obvious and natural decision. We have no time to lose. Does the choice now seem obvious to you too?

Confronted by life's daily challenges, we will forget to make this choice. We'll slide back into our old, habituated ways. To help safeguard against this inevitability, I think it can be helpful to write a contract outlining your commitment to your body, now *and* in the future. Title it "My Pledge to My Body."

To get you started, I'll give you an example of mine.

Dear body, I respect and honor you through thick and thin, through good times and bad, though health and illness. You don't have to do *anything, achieve* anything to be awarded my love. It is enough that you *are, and for that I adore you.*

You can adopt mine, if that feels good and right to you. Or you can write your own. Choose now. One way or another, grab your journal, and either copy mine verbatim on your own paper or write your new pledge now.

Good job! When you make this pledge to yourself now, and get going, *now,* you set yourself on a positive future trajectory for health of all parts of your self now and in the future.

Once we make the decision to stop defining ourselves through material descriptions, then we are free to stop forever the endless self-criticism about the body, instead reallocating that energy to other areas of our person and life. Your only belongings are your actions. Now that you've freed up the time and energy you've historically spent harassing the body, what are you going to *do* with it? What actions do you want to take?

It matters most what we do today.

USE YOUR BODY TO FIND YOUR PURPOSE

Many people coach on living your best life, or finding your purpose, but few specifically use body-centric techniques to find answers. My assertion is twofold:

1. When we waste time thinking negatively about our bodies, we tie up energy that we could use otherwise in our lives, *and*

2. It is specifically through the body that we will arrive at an understanding of who we are and what we are here to do.

There's tremendous irony in this. Because you are what you do, how you spend your time is mission critical. By restoring our ownership of our female bodies, our understanding of what they are, and our confidence in their magic, we have access to better answers for these questions:

- What are you?

- What are you here to do?

Knowledge of our own bodies makes us smarter in ways that benefit us immensely.

- We can take better care of our own health, healing, self-care, and wellness through practical understanding and intuitive insight.

- We can use our bodies to access otherwise unavailable knowledge and wisdom about ourselves, others, and the world.

The body is our radio antenna to the divine. But we can't use it to answer these questions when we judge and abuse it. The answer to *What are you here to do?* won't come to you honestly and truthfully through merely thinking while excluding your body from the process. The answer will come to you through creating a healthy, daily relationship with it, feeling the question with all parts of your body, and opening your awareness to answers from the beyond. I believe that each of us was put here on earth with a divine mission. It may be simple, humble, and small. It may be complex and grandiose. Both of these—and everything in between!—are valid and sacred duties.

The body is our radio antenna to the divine.

Additionally, when you trust your body and it trusts you, an entirely new layer of healing energy becomes available. By healing, I mean doing your own internal work of personal transformation so that you and your energies are fully available to you and the world. The way Frida Kahlo did. She transformed the suffering of her life into great beauty.

Change can take a long time, and sometimes it appears like an overwhelming or impossible challenge. When you see others achieving change, it might appear simple because what *you* see, on the outside, is a quantum leap, when it actually took years of preparation to attain a growth spurt. My business coach has a saying—overnight successes are twenty years in the making. That's because it can sometimes take a very long time for our thoughts to manifest in the material world. Our thoughts are the very seeds of everything that we birth into the world. Because thoughts are energy, they can move fast, but physical matter moves much more slowly.

When I'm teaching yoga, one of the results that I like to share with my students is how my feet used to be painfully flat, but thanks to Forrest Yoga and a way of engaging the feet that we call "active feet" they now have arches. My rehabilitated feet began with an idea—the idea that *change is possible for me. I can change.* Without this notion we are stuck. It took about twenty years of belief, dedication, and determined work, but it happened!

When you think good thoughts about the body, trust it, give it the things that it needs to thrive, and honor its uniqueness and the sheer miracle of your existence, this puts you in a great place to uplevel your healing and access your life's work, using the body to retrieve the knowledge and wisdom within and beyond you.

Let's review the core practices from each lesson.

1. Create a central helpful thought.

2. Access your heart's desires daily with your heart log.

3. Create a sankalpah.

4. Use the Forrest Yoga Formula for Change.

5. Nourish your senses.

6. Take care of your unique body and delight your spirit with daily sadhana.

These practices, and a plentitude of other tips and exercises, are intended to help you clean up your thinking about your body so *it* can do its rightful, sacred task of connecting to the divine and your life's purpose.

Figuring out what you are here for will be a lifelong adventure. It will shift and change and evolve as you do. Sometimes I feel like I'm changing so very fast inside, it's hard to keep track of what I really think I am here for from day to day. This is the challenge of being a spirit in a material form. The inner *koshas* all move and change faster than a slow, stubborn body. Routine questioning for these answers helps us keep our finger on the pulse of our life force.

Here are three exercises to help you begin considering what you're here for and to use repeatedly as you begin to uncover answers.

Exercise #1: Brahmari Chakra Process

This process, which I learned from my teacher Ana Forrest, uses the body to help you gain insight and wisdom from it.

You might recall what the *chakras* are from Lesson 2, but let's review. The chakras ("wheels") are part of our "subtle body." *Koshas* create a map of the human body in layers, from obvious and "gross" to invisible and "subtle." I think of the koshas as lining up on an X axis. The chakras line up on a Y axis, like a radio tower that plugs the body into the ground and extends us into the sky. Anatomically, the chakras correspond with seven nerve plexuses positioned along the spine and into the skull. They're hubs of energetic activity in the both the physical and metaphysical bodies.

This is relevant to expanding your understanding of your own body in a mystical way.

On the physical body, the chakras cover these anatomical regions:

First chakra: Bottom of the pelvis

Second chakra: Belly button

Third chakra: Bottom of the ribs

Fourth chakra: Center of the chest

Fifth chakra: Throat

Sixth chakra: Between the eyebrows

Seventh chakra: Top of the skull

For those who like to visualize, each chakra has a corresponding color:

First chakra: Red

Second chakra: Orange

Third chakra: Yellow

Fourth chakra: Green and rose

Fifth chakra: Blue

Sixth chakra: Indigo

Seventh chakra: Violet

If you visualize the seven chakras as two interlocking triangles, with the bottom one upright and the top one upside down, their points would interlock at the fourth, heart *chakra*. The triangles represent the two realms that a human being occupies—one is the material realm of the first three chakras, which govern elimination (first chakra), procreation (second chakra) and sustenance (third chakra). The other is the spiritual realm of the upper triangle; the upper three chakras govern wisdom (fifth chakra), spirituality (sixth chakra) and divinity (seventh chakra).

Next, *brahmari*: it means "to hum," and the brahmari pranayama (breathing exercise) is called "The Bee Buzzing Breath."

Hum right now. Can you feel which aspect of your body vibrates with your humming? Slide the pitch up. Now what part of the body is resonating with your voice? Check that your teeth are separated so that the jaw is relaxed and your lips vibrate, perhaps tickling one another. It should feel good! Relax your throat so that your humming doesn't irritate your vocal cords.

For this exercise, you will purposefully target aspects of your body with the buzzing of your voice.

Before you begin the process, choose a question to ask your body. Yes, you're going to *ask your body to help you with the circumstances of your life.* You talk to it all the time, anyway. This is just a new kind of conversation, one that honors the body's wisdom.

Each chakra governs its own basic issues. Anodea Judith describes them like this:

1.   Survival

2.   Sexuality

3.   Power

4.   Love

5.   Communication

6.   Intuition

7.   Cognition[57]

Medical intuitive and mystic Carlolyn Myss believes the chakras are the sites of our dark passions and also our graces.

1.   Pride/Reverence

2.   Avarice/Piety

3.   Luxury/Understanding

4.   Wrath/Fortitude

5.   Gluttony/Counsel

6.   Envy/Knowledge

7.   Sloth/Wisdom[58]

As you go through this process of engaging your chakras in a question from your life, know that they contain wisdom on these topics.

For this process, you'll need

•   About twenty minutes free time

•   Your journal

•   Somewhere comfortable to sit and make noise, uninterrupted

- A question into which you would appreciate insight from your body

Got that? Then you're ready to begin!

1. Put your hands on top of your head, at your seventh chakra. Use your voice to buzz the top of your head! Give it five to eight buzzy breaths. As you do so, hold your question in mind. If you get any information while doing this—a sensation, an image, a sound, a smell, or a taste (remember, the body doesn't speak English!)—pause and record this in your journal as information coming from the seventh chakra.

2. Put your hands around your eyes and ears, at your sixth chakra. Use your voice to vibrate this part of your body, holding your question in mind. Repeat the steps for the seventh chakra.

3. Place your hands at your throat, at the fifth chakra, and repeat the same steps.

4. Place your hands on your heart center, the fourth chakra, and repeat the steps.

5. Place your hands at your bottom ribs, at the third chakra, and repeat the steps.

6. Put one hand on your low belly and one hand over your sacrum, the bony triangle at the bottom of your spine between the sides of your pelvis, the second chakra. Repeat the steps.

7. Put fingers of one hand on your pubic bone and fingers of the other hand on you tailbone, at the first chakra. Repeat the instructions.

When you're done with all seven chakras, you may feel called to go back and communicate with one again. Do that! The final step is to decide how you can take action on what you've learned. What is something you can do soon, if not today?

I love this process because it calls up the truth that our bodies contain wisdom of their own. Mostly, we never have this important conversation with our bodies, and therefore miss the insights they could offer on, well, everything!

After doing the brahmari chakra process, you might have information you didn't before that you can now apply to Exercise #2, What's My Mission? If you look at the exercise and feel like you're drawing a blank, make that question the topic of the brahmari chakra process or your next meditation. The question would be: *What am I here to do with this one precious life?*

Exercise #2: What's My Mission?

List five reasons you think you might be here, on earth. Your mission. Your raison d'être. Your purpose. Don't think too hard, just flow. You could make this question the topic of a movement practice!

Exercise #3: A Perfect Day

My music mentor once said to me, "It all comes down to how you want to spend the minutes of your day." How do you want to spend the minutes and seconds of your life? If all we have is *now*, this is a crucial question! This moment is all we are assured of.

Describe a perfect, idyllic day, one in which, in every moment, you feel happy with how you are spending your time. Imagine that this day is yours to enjoy every day of your life moving forward. How would you describe that day? Do it in the greatest amount of detail that you can, with descriptions that satisfy all of the senses and all aspects of your being.

You can repeat these exercises daily, monthly, yearly! You can perform them in a ritual, with movement so that you can engage your body more directly in the moment of questioning. But the more you repair your relationship with the body and become increasingly embodied, experiencing a steadily improving daily baseline, the greater the access you will have to the body's wisdom without needing to do something elaborate or specific to "get embodied."

In this lesson, we've tied together some of the big elements from all the lessons while at the same time continuing to grow our understanding of what we are, materially and ethereally. The main conundrum of being human is that we are and are *not* our bodies. I believe that what we've perceived as the obstacle to our happiness (the body) is in fact *the way* to our greatest fruition as humans. Our bodies are, truthfully, the very tool we must rely on most to evolve into the people we're most meant to be: our higher selves.

As women, we've been educated that our bodies are the wrong bodies, and because of our sex we've been systematically excluded from most of the spiritual and religious experiences of antiquity and of modernity. But it is precisely our bodies that will bring us to a conclusive understanding of our selves, who we are, and what we're here for, *no matter what*, and perhaps *exactly because of what* they've endured in life—injury, abuse, illness, pregnancy, childbirth, aging—*whatever!* The past hasn't been kind to women or our bodies, and in many instances we've cooperated in absorbing, sustaining, and spreading wrongful ideas about ourselves. The key to undoing this history lies in how we think about ourselves, speak about ourselves, and behave toward ourselves and others. And now, you are in possession of the tools you need to accomplish just that! This book is a manual detailing exactly *how*.

We are so lucky to be alive right now. History is happening and it's ours to make! The future is, indeed, female. Change is afoot, and we have better personal resources than ever before in the history of the human species. But please join me in making sure we responsibly manifest *the very best* aspects of humanity, by adopting the many mind-set shifts you've learned in this book. When you use these helpful replacement mind-sets to shift away from your garden of dark thoughts, you're awakening and stepping onto the path of light. Let's *be* the future we most desire. How? Embody the best aspects of humanity, and live out our highest calling, for the good of all and harm to none. This is how we manifest heaven on earth. I look forward to standing in the light alongside you, sisters and brothers! An army of angels, we shall be.

You're On Your Way

Dearest reader—congratulations! You've arrived at the end of this book, *this transformational journey,* which I hope has delivered you to the threshold of a wonderful new world, one where you spend far less time doing things that don't actually matter that much and far more time engaged in activities you love with people you care about, and where your body plays a new, healthy central role in all of your life, rather than existing as an object of derision; a world in which your body is your foremost ally on the path of self-discovery.

Know, too, that your decisions will positively affect the people around you, and you may in fact become a role model for body acceptance, confidence, and appreciation. Some people may chafe against this new you. Don't worry! It's not *your* job to change their minds (remember how hard that is, anyway?). It's your job to be *you.* Unflinchingly. Authentically. Powerfully. *Radically.* No matter what may come. And it's not your job to be overly concerned with what others think about you. Become wise about the impact you have on people, and choose your actions to orchestrate the best outcomes for all. Over time, people may come around once they see how your integrity and the changes you've made alter the landscape of your life for the better.

At the end of this book, you may still feel dissatisfaction with your body. That's okay. The course outlined in this book isn't intended to be another thing for you to "get right" or fail (or succeed!) with. It's simply additional information. In my experience, body dissatisfaction is something that's with us for the long haul, even as it improves. If you feel into yourself, can you detect some change, any change at all? Has your tolerance for weight gain increased? Do you spend even 1 percent less time concerned over your appearance? Have you begun calling in sick when you are? Do you sleep more? Chances are you've made *some* small change. Small things become big things, over time.

Think of an oak tree. Once upon a time, it was a tiny acorn.

If you cannot honestly identify a change in yourself—still, no worries. Rest assured, you have been changed by the act of reading this book from cover to cover. If reading it didn't mean something to you, you would have put it down long ago. Know that this change in your self-confidence and your life is going to show up. You won't know when or where, but it's coming. So breathe easy. All is coming. And it's entirely possible it will be far better than you could have possibly imagined.

Small things become big things, over time.

Above all, no matter the immediate or long-term outcomes, I hope that you can feel good about yourself for being brave-hearted and persisting in your own journey of self-discovery and transformation. You might not feel it every day, but yours is a heroic journey. In the stories, heroic journeys are the best kind. And the ending isn't where the juicy stuff occurs—it's everything along the way. The lows are where the *really* good stuff happens. Just remember that! In your darkest moments, remember *that.*

So congratulate yourself for being on the best kind of journey, and think of others who have as well (for me, Frida Kahlo is one of them), and all the goodness and beauty they added to the world. That's you! A peaceful warrior. An earth angel. Before you brush that off as impossible, just stop. What if you were, indeed, a peaceful warrior? What if you were put here on this earth to bring goodness and true beauty into it? I hold that vision for you and for all women. Let's hold it together!

The point of life is to live. Wake up, and live your life!

I'm terrible at goodbyes. So I'll just say, I sincerely hope to see you, in person, somewhere soon. Yoga, anyone?

Blessings, and—bye for now!

Erica

P.S. Be sure to check the Resource Guide! There's a bonus meditation in there for you! ;-)

Acknowledgments

I must begin by expressing my thanks to my students and clients in New York City and around the world. Yes, you. Put your name here. Teaching you and spending time with you is the manifestation of my life's work, my truest joy, and the source of my own learning. Thank you for allowing me to be of service to you.

To Jackie Summers, who saw the very beginnings of this material and heard in it, a book. Thank you for encouraging me to write. Thank you, Ana Forrest, for the magic of Forrest Yoga; for teaching me about embodiment, seeing me, and being my friend. To Linda Loewenthal, who read my blogs and heard a fresh new voice: thank you for your time and support, and for guiding me to some of the next people mentioned here. To my agent, Coleen O'Shea, whose signoff "Onward!" has come to signify to me a mind-set of its own and one I've adopted. Thank you for your patience and interest in this project. To Linda Sivertsen, who has become a friend and spiritual guide along the birthing process of this book. Thank you for believing in me and calling to check in and make sure that I didn't just let the book wither on the vine. To my first editor, Ryan Buresh, who sent me an email out of the blue, and whose dedication to developing the project has ushered it to publication with New Harbinger. To my other editor, Jennifer Holder, whose eye for, well, *everything* has made this a better book, many times over! To Kristi Hein, who bled my manuscript of possibly *thousands* of commas and made so many sentences read more smoothly.

Thank you, Sharon Lynch, for helping me handle editorial crises of the personal kind, and Lori Edelman, for listening to me despair and always, always relentlessly being the adult. Thank you, Ann Conrad, for being my friend for life. Thank you, Kirsten Collins, for being the voice of reason amidst so much craziness and for helping me make sense of New York existence. Thank you, Devi, for your reparenting. Thank you, Isaac, Karim, Eduardo, Vic, Dave, Benjamin, Jason, all the good men around me, and an assortment of friends who have reached out to ask "How's the book going?" or just to check on me. Thank you, Maria Bassett, for being my right-hand woman. I know I'm hard to wrangle. Thank you, Les Thimmig, for always encouraging me, no matter if it took me away from our pursuits together. You've been a source and an inspiration of "unconditional love."

Finally, and perhaps most importantly, thank you O.U.T. and cousins. All of you, but especially Anna, Whit, and Cary for loving me. And thank you, Cary, for being my *prima Hermana*.

I love you all! Onward!

Resource Guide

The Adore Your Body Telesummit (the best of them!)
http://www.ericamather.com/adoreyourbodytelesummitbest

The Adore Your Body 3-Part Training, addressing some common questions.
http://www.ericamather.com/3-part-training

Accessible Yoga: a nonprofit organization working to ensure yoga access for everyone.
http://www.accessibleyoga.org

Roxane Gay, author, professor, and speaker.
http://www.roxanegay.com

The Body Positive Institute: a nonprofit organization that educates on the topic of body image and body positivity in schools and communities.
http://www.thebodypositive.org

The Beacon Program: mastery over food and disordered eating.
http://www.beaconprogram.com

Cuddlist, for getting more human contact into your life, from safe, certified providers.
http://www.cuddlist.com

DoTerra, for great essential oils.
https://my.doterra.com/musesproductioninc

Health at Every Size, for understanding that "healthy" looks and feels many different ways.
https://haescommunity.com

Jes Baker: author, speaker, and blogger on body autonomy, self-love, and mental health.
http://www.themilitantbaker.com

Dr. Betty Martin, for understanding touch—receiving and giving.
http://www.bettymartin.org/videos

The Moon Deck, "an interactive tool for connecting to your intuition and emotional health through the path of self-love and ritual."
http://www.themoondeck.com

Sonya Renee Taylor, author of the bestselling book, *The Body is Not an Apology: The Power of Radical Self-Love.*
http://www.thebodyisnotanapology.com

We Are the Real Deal: an educational blog for today's youth.
http://www.wearetherealdeal.com

Virgie Tovar, author and activist.
http://www.virgietovar.com

Audio: A guided meditation to help you get to know your body.
http://www.newharbinger.com/43430

Endnotes

1   Thích Nhất Hạnh, "The Art of Mindful Living," read by the author (Louisville, KY: Sounds True, 1999).

2   Kathleen Kennedy Townsend, "The Pursuit of Happiness: What the Founders Meant—And Didn't," *Atlantic,* June 20, 2011, https://www.theatlantic.com/business/archive/2011/06/the -pursuit-of-happiness-what-the-founders-meant-and-didnt/240708/.

3   Ibid.

4   Jon Clifton, "Mood of the World Upbeat on International Happiness Day," *GALLUP,* March 19, 2015, http://news.gallup.com /poll/182009/mood-world-upbeat-international-happiness-day.aspx.

5   Robert F. Kennedy, remarks at the University of Kansas, March 18, 1968.

6   Oliver Burkeman, *The Antidote: Happiness for People Who Can't Stand Positive Thinking* (New York: Faber and Faber, 2012), 6–7.

7   Pema Chödrön, *The Places That Scare You: A Guide to Fearless- ness in Difficult Times* (Boulder, CO: Shambala, 2002), 38–39.

8   Robert Greene, *The 48 Laws of Power* (New York: Penguin Books, 2000), 405.

9   Geshe Michael Roach and Lama Christie McNally, *The Diamond Cutter: The Buddha on Managing Your Business and Your Life* (New York: Doubleday, 2009), 88.

10   Daniele LaPorte, "The Declaration of Deserving Just Because You're Here" (n.d.), http://www.daniellelaporte.com/the -declaration-of-deserving-just-because-youre-here/.

11   Danielle LaPorte, "How to Wish Someone Well for Real in a Way That Will Blow Your Heart Wide Open" (n.d.), http://www .daniellelaporte.com/how-to-wish-someone-well-for-real-in-a-way -that-will-blow-your-heart-wide-open/.

12   Greene, *The 48 Laws of Power.*

13   Virgie Tovar, "Dear Virgie: What's the History of Diet Culture?" *Wear Your Voice,* February 23, 2016, https://wearyourvoicemag.com/body-politics/dear-virgie-whats-history-diet-culture.

14   Ibid.

15   W. G. Parrot and R. H. Smith, "Distinguishing the Experiences of Envy and Jealousy," *Journal of Personality and Social Psychology* 64 (1993): 906–920.

16   Paulo Coelho, *The Alchemist* (New York: Harper One, 2014).

17   Brené Brown, *I Thought It Was Just Me (But It Isn't): Making the Journey From "What Will People Think?" to "I Am Enough"* (New York: Gotham Books, 2008), 96.

18   Thích Nhất Hạnh, *Understanding Our Mind: 50 Verses on Buddhist Psychology* (Berkeley, CA: Parallax Press, 2002).

19   The MoonDeck, www.themoondeck.com.

20   Naomi Wolf, *The Beauty Myth : How Images of Beauty Are Used Against Women* (New York: Harper Perennial, 2002).

21   Roach and McNally, *The Diamond Cutter,* 40.

22   Thích Nhất Hạnh, *Teachings on Love,* 23–34.

23   Jeffery Kluger and Alexandra Sifferlin, "How to Live Longer, Better (You're Still Going to Die, Though)," *Time,* February 26, 2018, 47.

24   Ana Forrest, *Fierce Medicine: Breakthrough Practices to Heal the Body and Ignite the Spirit* (New York: HarperOne, 2012), 46.

25   Portia Nelson, *There's a Hole in My Sidewalk: The Romance of Self-Discovery* (Los Angeles, CA: Popular Library, 1977).

26   Silvia Federici, *Caliban and the Witch: Women, the Body, and Primitive Accumulation* (Brooklyn, NY: Autonomedia, 2004), 47.

27   T. Christian Miller, ProPublica, and Ken Armstrong, The Marshall Project, "An Unbelievable Story of Rape," ProPublica, December 16, 2015, https://www.propublica.org/article/false-rape-accusations-an-unbelievable-story.

28   Federici, *Caliban and the Witch,* 135.

29   Ibid., 184.

30   Ibid., 139.

31   Ibid., 138.

32   Gary Taubes, *Why We Get Fat: And What to Do About It* (New York: Knopf, 2011).

33   Matthew Sanford, *Waking: A Memoir of Trauma and Transcendence* (Emmaus, PA: Rodale Books, 2008), 222.

34   Pema Chödrön, *The Places That Scare You,* 28.

35   Ibid.

36   Ibid.

37   Rupa Mehta, *The Nalini Method: 7 Workouts for 7 Moods* (Berkeley, CA: Seal Press, 2016).

38   Federici, *Caliban and the Witch,* 142.

39   Ibid., 142–143.

40   Linda Johnsen, "The Koshas: 5 Layers of Being" (n.d.), Yoga International, https://yogainternational.com/article/view/the-koshas-5-layers-of-being.

41   Visit http://www.nationaleatingdisorders.org for immediate support and to find a treatment provider near you.

42   Anahad O'Connor, "When We Eat, or Don't Eat, May Be Critical for Health," *New York Times,* July 24, 2018, https://www.nytimes.com/2018/07/24/well/when-we-eat-or-dont-eat-may-be-critical-for-health.html?hp&action=click&pgtype=Homepage&clickSource=story-heading&module=second-column-region&region=top-news&WT.nav=top-news.

43   Ibid.

44   Michael Moss, "The Extraordinary Science of Addictive Junk Food," *New York Times,* February 20, 2013, https://www.nytimes.com/2013/02/24/magazine/the-extraordinary-science-of-junk-food.html.

45   Michael Moss, "How The Food Industry Helps Engineer Our Cravings," interview by Jeremy Hobson, *Here & Now* series "America on the Scale," National Public Radio, December 16, 2015, https://www.npr.org/sections/thesalt/2015/12/16/459981099/how-the-food-industry-helps-engineer-our-cravings.

46   Camila Domonoske, "50 Years Ago, Sugar Industry Quietly Paid Scientists to Point Blame at Fat," National Public Radio, September 13, 2016, https://www.npr.org/sections/thetwo-way/2016/09/13/493739074/50-years-ago-sugar-industry-quietly-paid-scientists-to-point-blame-at-fat.

47   Centers for Disease Control, "1 in 3 Adults Don't Get Enough Sleep," February 18, 2016, https://www.cdc.gov/media/releases/2016/p0215-enough-sleep.html.

48   Sleep Academy, "Sleep and Sickness: Tips to Better Rest," http://sleepacademy.org/category/sleep-your-health/.

49   Taubes, *Why We Get Fat,* 43.

50   Ibid., 47.

51   http://www.cuddlist.com.

52   Virgie Tovar, *You Have the Right to Remain Fat* (New York: First Feminist Press, 2018), 73.

53   Pema Chödrön, *The Places That Scare You,* 130.

54   Roach and McNally, *The Diamond Cutter,* 213.

55   Thích Nhất Hạnh, *Breathe: A Thích Nhất Hạnh Journal* (Berkeley, CA: Parallax Press, 2011).

56   Thích Nhất Hạnh, "The Art of Mindful Living" (Disc 2).

57   Anodea Judith, *Wheels of Life: A User's Guide to the Chakra System* (Woodbury, MN: Llewellyn Publications, 2006).

58   Caroline Myss, *Defy Gravity: Healing Beyond the Bounds of Reason* (New York: Hay House, 2009).

Erica Mather is a lifelong teacher who has struggled with emotional overeating, compulsive overexercising, and body dysmorphia disorder. As an embodiment educator, she guides people to feel better in, and about, their bodies. Her Adore Your Body Transformational Programs help overcome body image challenges, and The Yoga Clinic of New York City helps students, teachers, and health professionals to learn about empowered self-care for the body. Mather is a recognized body image expert, a Forrest Yoga lineage-holder, and was also named one of the next generation's important yoga teachers by *Yoga Journal*. She writes for *mindbodygreen* on the topic of body image challenges, is a regular columnist for *Rivertown Magazine*, and is a popular repeat interview on the *SoulFeed Podcast*, Hay House Radio's Angel Club, and many more. Mather lives in New York City, NY. Visit her at www.ericamather.com.

Real change *is* possible

For more than forty-five years, New Harbinger has published proven-effective self-help books and pioneering workbooks to help readers of all ages and backgrounds improve mental health and well-being, and achieve lasting personal growth. In addition, our spirituality books offer profound guidance for deepening awareness and cultivating healing, self-discovery, and fulfillment.

Founded by psychologist Matthew McKay and Patrick Fanning, New Harbinger is proud to be an independent, employee-owned company. Our books reflect our core values of integrity, innovation, commitment, sustainability, compassion, and trust. Written by leaders in the field and recommended by therapists worldwide, New Harbinger books are practical, accessible, and provide real tools for real change.

newharbingerpublications

MORE BOOKS

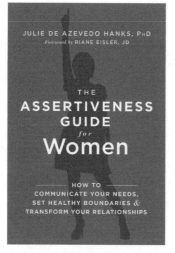
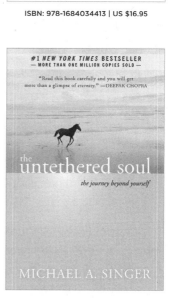
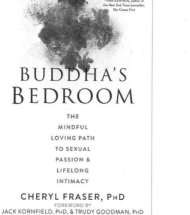
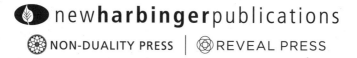

Register your **new harbinger** titles for additional benefits!

When you register your **new harbinger** title—purchased in any format, from any source—you get access to benefits like the following:

- Downloadable accessories like printable worksheets and extra content

- Instructional videos and audio files

- Information about updates, corrections, and new editions

Not every title has accessories, but we're adding new material all the time.

Access free accessories in 3 easy steps:

1. Sign in at NewHarbinger.com (or **register** to create an account).

2. Click on **register a book**. Search for your title and click the **register** button when it appears.

3. Click on the **book cover or title** to go to its details page. Click on **accessories** to view and access files.

That's all there is to it!

If you need help, visit:

NewHarbinger.com/accessories

new harbinger
CELEBRATING
40 YEARS